D1088933

COMPUTED TOMOGRAPHY TECHNOLOGY

EUCLID SEERAM, R.T., B.Sc.

British Columbia Institute of Technology
Burnaby, British Columbia

with contributions by

THOMAS PAYNE, Ph.D.

Abbott Northwestern Hospital
Minneapolis, Minnesota

RC
78.7
.T6
S37
1982

1982

W. B. SAUNDERS COMPANY

Philadelphia / London / Toronto / Mexico City
Rio de Janeiro / Sydney / Tokyo

W. B. Saunders Company: West Washington Square
Philadelphia, PA   19105

1 St. Anne's Road
Eastbourne, East Sussex BN21 3UN, England

1 Goldthorne Avenue
Toronto, Ontario M8Z 5T9, Canada

Apartado 26370 – Cedro 512
Mexico 4, D.F., Mexico

Rua Coronel Cabrita, 8
Sao Cristovao Caixa Postal 21176
Rio de Janeiro, Brazil

9 Waltham Street
Artarmon, N.S.W. 2064, Australia

Ichibancho, Central Bldg., 22-1 Ichibancho
Chiyoda-Ku, Tokyo 102, Japan

INDIANA
UNIVERSITY LIBRARY

JUL 18 1983

NORTHWEST

Library of Congress Cataloging in Publication Data

Seeram, Euclid.

Computed tomography technology.

1. Tomography.   I. Payne, Thomas, 1944–   II. Title
   [DNLM: 1. Tomography, X-ray computed – Methods.
   WN 160 S453c]

RC78.7.T6S37   616.07'572   81–48093

ISBN 0-7216-8059-3   AACR2

INDIANA
UNIVERSITY
NORTHWEST

LIBRARY

Computed Tomography Technology   ISBN   0-7216-8059-3

© 1982 by W. B. Saunders Company. Copyright under the Uniform Copyright Convention.
Simultaneously published in Canada. All rights reserved. This book is protected by copyright.
No part of it may be reproduced, stored in a retrieval system, or transmitted in any form or by any
means, electronic, mechanical, photocopying, recording, or otherwise, without written permission
from the publisher. Made in the United States of America. Press of W. B. Saunders Company.
Library of Congress catalog card number 81-48093.

Last digit is the print number: 9   8   7   6   5   4   3   2   1

rJ
7-15-83

*This book is dedicated with love
to my wife Trish
and son David,
two of my life treasures.*

CT FOREWORD

Radiology has just emerged from a period of technological renaissance. In 1972, a new method of taking x-ray pictures was introduced by G. N. Hounsfield (physicist) and J. Ambrose (neuroradiologist). They had just completed testing of the first clinical computed tomographic (CT) scanner. For the remainder of the decade, CT was in the limelight as a rapidly developing but costly example of medical technology.

Today, CT scanning is considered to be an essential and accepted part of standard radiologic practice in most large hospitals. CT scans of the head, body, or spine are considered essential in the proper diagnosis and management of patient disorders. It is important that those of us working in radiology know the tools of our trade. This book examines CT as an important tool in diagnostic radiologic imaging. The basic principles of CT operation, including computer fundamentals, are covered. Complex aspects of CT are reduced to understandable terminology. Euclid Seeram has done a good job of condensing and extracting pertinent information from the prolific CT literature.

J. Thomas Payne, Ph.D.

CT PREFACE

Computed tomography (CT) is now becoming recognized as one of the major branches of diagnostic radiology. It marks the beginning of a new activity for radiologists, technologists, medical physicists, and other related health professionals.

Ever since computed tomography was introduced into clinical radiology, there has been an increasing demand for textbooks on the fundamental principles of CT that present a solid foundation by introducing elementary theoretical groundwork and at the same time raise the reader's sophistication in the field as quickly and easily as possible. In considering these essentials, the purpose of this text is threefold: (1) To provide a clear and comprehensive introduction to the physical principles of CT through a discussion of the basic elements of computer technology and physico-mathematical concepts as they relate to CT. (2) To assist the reader in acquiring further understanding of the structure of CT. (3) To enable the reader to begin building a new vocabulary that will allow him to understand the literature pertaining to CT.

Having these objectives in mind, the text is intended for use in the following ways: (a) As a text for introductory courses in CT at the associate and baccalaureate degree levels, to be used either alone or with readings in the CT classics. (b) As an introductory reference text for professional radiologic personnel. (c) As a supplementary text for courses in applied fields, the purpose of which is to introduce the reader to the language of CT for use in applications to his field (e.g., biomedical technology). (d) As a guide to independent study. (e) As a rapid survey and review of important issues presented in introductory courses.

I have purposely written the book in a brief and concise manner to ensure that the reader's interest and attention are maintained, since the language of CT is relatively new. The text differs from others in that it is perhaps one of the first attempts to bring together the complex theory of CT and its clinical components at a rather elementary level, while still maintaining a certain degree of structure that promotes abstract thinking. Equally important, it contains summaries of key elements, review questions, and a small, selected bibliography, the purpose of which is to provide motivation and help the reader in the learning process.

Chapter 1 presents a general overview of the computer with respect to the basic components and operating principles. Computer applications in radiology are discussed briefly.

The principles of CT are introduced in Chapter 2 in terms of historical background, physical basis, and technology. Chapter 3 deals with a number of important features of the detection system in CT, x-ray sources, and collimation.

Chapter 4 lends itself to an introduction to mathematical techniques used in image reconstruction from projections without the use of rigorous mathematics.

A description of CT not only involves a discussion of physical principles but definitely warrants a description and identification of the equipment and components. Such treatment is given in Chapter 5.

In Chapter 6, several concepts relating to image quality are introduced and several factors influencing resolution are discussed.

Since dose in CT is of great concern to the physician and radiologic personnel, it is discussed in Chapter 7.

Although the text is physically oriented, I have included in Chapter 8 a discussion of some clinical aspects of CT for the purpose of completeness. Such aspects relate to efficacy, indications, patient preparation and positioning, and so on.

Finally, Chapter 9 presents an examination of future trends in CT, including essential economic considerations.

Throughout the text, I present the results of selected research findings under separate subsections. In presenting these findings, a number of direct quotations will be used so as not to detract from the original meaning. The results of these studies are important, since they lead to the establishment of standards, the implementation of safety procedures, and other related matters. It is my belief that the inclusion of these studies will serve to provide the student with information on some current areas of research, to open up new horizons for further discussion and perhaps investigation, and to enhance the general scope of the text.

In organizing and writing this text, I have assumed that the student has had a knowledge of basic radiologic physics; however, certain concepts (e.g., radiation attenuation) can be explained at a satisfactory depth by the instructor.

It is also my growing conviction that you will enjoy the pages that follow. Good luck in your pursuit of a new technology.

EUCLID SEERAM
British Columbia, Canada

ACKNOWLEDGMENTS

The material in this book represents what I believe to be a fairly comprehensive review of the literature on computed tomography. The real authors are those scientists, engineers, radiologists, and many others who have done the original research. In this regard I should like to express my sincere appreciation to Dr. G. N. Hounsfield, Nobel Prize winner, who made the technique clinically feasible. I should also like to thank him for his biographic data and portrait and for his permission to use them in this text.

The book had its inception at the Ottawa General Hospital School of Radiography with a series of notes given to student radiologic technologists, who elicited a few rather important concerns that resulted in a number of additions to the text material.
further at the British Columbia Institute of Technology and resulted in a formal 12-week course for graduate technologists. I am grateful to these students, who elicited a few rather important concerns that resulted in a number of additions to the text material.

Two teachers have influenced my early years in radiography and my further educational development, and I owe them my special thanks. They are Sr. M. York, S.C.O., R.T., a warm and caring individual who provided my first experience in teaching computed tomography, and C. Hebert, Ph.D., to whom I owe my understanding of radiologic physics. One other teacher to whom I am also grateful is Professor M. B. Fenton, Ph.D., of Carleton University in Ottawa, whose course on biology taught me the rudiments of technical writing and reporting and the elements of archival research.

The book would not have been possible without the efforts of a great number of people. I therefore express thanks to all the authors, publishers, and CT equipment manufacturers who not only furnished information but gave their willing permission to reproduce data and illustrations in the text. I would especially like to acknowledge the help of General Electric Company, Medical Systems Division; EMI Medical, Inc.; Ohio Nuclear; Pfizer, Inc.; and Picker International. One other company that deserves mention here is I.B.M., which supplied a good deal of information on computers and provided the photographs used in Chapter 1.

It is my pleasure to mention the individuals whose efforts contributed to this project. The works on computed tomography by E. C. McCullough,

Ph.D., of the Mayo Clinic, and J. T. Payne, Ph.D., Abbott Northwestern Hospital, provided the basic framework used in planning this text. Their research publications have been cited a number of times in this book. I should like especially to extend my sincere thanks and appreciation to Dr. J. Thomas Payne, medical physicist, for his contribution of the chapter on Radiation Dose and for his excellent review of the entire manuscript. His comments, suggestions, and corrections have been invaluable. Others include R. A. Brooks, Ph.D., National Institutes of Health; R. K. Cacak, Ph.D., University of Colorado Health Sciences Center; G. Cohen, Ph.D., University of Texas Health Sciences Center at Houston; S. J. Riederer, physicist, University of Wisconsin, Medical Physics Division; E. Ritman, M.D., Ph.D., Head, Biodynamics Research Unit, Mayo Clinic; C. M. Strother, M.D., University of Wisconsin Clinical Sciences Center; D. P. Boyd, Ph.D., University of California; G. A. Hay, Department of Medical Physics, University of Leeds; and Susan Weber, supervisor of CT scanning, Cleveland Clinic.

I owe thanks to A. Burgess, Ph.D., physicist in diagnostic radiology, University of British Columbia, who provided answers to several of my questions on computed tomography, and to Mark Dumont, M.Sc., computer specialist, who reviewed Chapter 1 and provided useful comments that helped to bring the chapter to its present form.

I must also express my gratitude to Bev Brown and Shirley Matkowski, CT technologists, who assisted me with some clinical details for Chapter 8.

My friend and colleague Norma Smith, R.T., B.A., Program Head, Radiography Section, British Columbia Institute of Technology, deserves special mention here. Her fitting disposition and concern helped me to maintain the impetus necessary to complete this task. In this regard also, I should like to thank L. Timko, M.D., radiologist, whose thoughtfulness and attitude gave me encouragement.

To all the people at Saunders who were involved in the making of this text, I owe a good deal of thanks. I would like to identify particularly Marie Low, former editor, Allied Health Sciences, whose enthusiasm and dynamic professionalism set the proposed manuscript into motion. Her comments and guidance were extremely helpful and encouraging. Wendy Phillips, former assistant editor, Allied Health Sciences, also provided encouragement and assistance in reshaping the manuscript to bring it to its present form. Baxter Venable, Medical Editor, supervised the completion of this project and provided constant feedback on various aspects of its development. I would also like to acknowledge the Editorial/Design/Production Team at Saunders for their meticulous work on the general layout of the manuscript.

Finally, my family's encouragement and help is what really brought the text to its present form. My wife, Trish, a very special person, provided the motivation throughout the research and writing stages of this book. She influenced and also contributed to my professional and educational development, particularly my university studies, and I am most appreciative of all her support in this undertaking, and for her help in the galley and page proof stages of publication. To my son David, a very perceptive and special lad, who gave me the "good feelings" about the project throughout all aspects of its development — thanks, pal.

Last, but not least, I thank my barber-stylist, Lyle Folkett, a well-read gentleman who wanted to know more about computed tomography.

CT A NOTE TO THE STUDENT

To assist you in the study of this text, each chapter is preceded by an outline and concludes with a summary of the main points. Such an outline is to guide you into the material, while the summary will indicate to you whether you have grasped the concepts.

The following suggestions are offered to enable you to achieve the general objectives of the text:

a. Consider Chapter 1 a very important chapter. It must not be skipped over, since the computer is now a key element in diagnostic radiology.

b. Consider Chapter 2 a pivotal chapter, since it is the basis of this text. It should be referred to as often as necessary to ensure understanding of further concepts.

c. Read the appropriate chapter before each lecture. This initial reading is intended to provide you with the content and language of the course.

d. After studying each chapter, read through the summary section to review the important points in the chapter.

e. To ensure that the main points have been assimilated, complete the review questions.

f. It is highly recommended that you read through the selected reading material as a basis for further discussion and insight into CT.

CT CONTENTS

CTINTRODUCTION

Innovations are quite commonplace in twentieth-century society. More specifically, innovations are becoming commonplace in the radiology department. New methods, ideas, and techniques, and hence new equipment, are constantly being generated so that improved patient care and optimum diagnostic information can be acquired.

As an important technological development, the rate of growth of the computer industry is increasing because of the numerous new possibilities for analysis and information processing. The computer has arrived in the radiology department, and its applications are receiving widespread attention.

The introduction of the computer in radiology goes back two decades. In 1955, K. C. Tsien used the computer to provide rapid and accurate calculations of radiation dose distributions in cancer patients. As his problem was a mathematical one, the use of the computer proved fruitful. This created a stimulus for other workers, and hence a series of applications was generated.

Today, computer applications in radiology range from the automated handling of patient records and radiologic reporting to difficult problems in imaging. Imaging applications include computer aided diagnosis, automated image analysis, and computed tomography. Computed tomography (CT) is a new imaging modality that was developed in 1969 by Godfrey N. Hounsfield of Electric and Musical Industries (EMI), Limited, a British-based international group of companies.

In CT, special detectors are used to measure x-rays passing through an object. This information is then sent to a computer, which reconstructs an image of the object by using complex mathematical techniques. The image is displayed on a television screen for viewing and photographic recording. It can also be obtained as a numerical print-out in which the numbers are the relative absorption values of the internal structures of the object.

In 1967, Hounsfield was investigating pattern recognition techniques when he deduced that if an x-ray beam were passed through a body from all directions and if measurements were made of all these x-ray transmissions, it would be possible to obtain information about the internal structure of that body. It was decided that this information should be presented to the radiologist in the form of pictures that would show three-dimensional representations of the part under examination.

The initial reconstruction of an image was simply based on multiple sampling to obtain multiple solutions. Since each part of the x-ray beam that

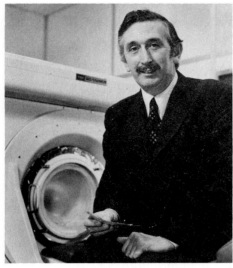

G. N. Hounsfield. (Courtesy of EMI Limited Central Research Laboratories, England.)

passed through the object formed a series of simultaneous equations, the use of a computer for this task was almost mandatory. Using a suitable mathematical model, the computer was programmed to reconstruct an image.

With encouragement from the British Department of Health to investigate the clinical feasibility of the technique, an apparatus was constructed, using radiation from a gamma source. Because of the low radiation output, the apparatus took about nine days to generate a picture. The computer took two and one-half hours to process the readings and had to solve 28,000 simultaneous equations. Various modifications were made and the study was then done using x-rays. The results were much more accurate, but it took about one day to produce a picture.

To evaluate the usefulness of such a machine, Dr. James Ambrose, a consultant radiologist at Atkinson-Morley's Hospital in Wimbledon, joined the study. Together, Hounsfield and Ambrose made readings from a specimen of human brain. The findings were rewarding, in that tumor tissue was differentiated from gray and white matter. Controlled experiments using "fresh bullocks' brains" showed details such as ventricles and the pineal gland. Experiments were also done using kidney sections from pigs.

In September, 1971, the first CT scanner was installed at Atkinson-Morley's Hospital, and under the direction of Dr. Ambrose clinical tests were conducted. The processing time for each picture was reduced to about 20 minutes. Some time later, with the utilization of minicomputers, the processing time for each picture was reduced even further to four and one-half minutes.

So remarkable is the CT that in many cases it generates a dramatic increase in diagnostic information over conventional x-ray techniques. In trying to describe its significance, one may be tempted to use the term "diagnostic breakthrough."

The introduction of CT in diagnostic radiology has been received with much enthusiasm. The first EMI CT scanner was restricted to brain imaging studies only, but researchers quickly adapted this technique for other parts of the body. Hence, new CT equipment has now become available to provide body scans with excellent resolution and contrast and with short scan times to minimize motion distortion. Other refinements of the first CT scanner have also been made with regard to scanning, the detection system, degrees of rotation, slice thickness, the number of readings, and so on. So rapid are these developments that already CT is in the so-called "fourth generation" of its history.

The fundamental concepts of CT can be traced back to numerous mathematical and other related developments. The history of reconstruction techniques began in 1917. A summary of other events is shown below:

1917	Radon	Laid down roots of tomography in terms of mathematics.
1956	Bracewell	Performed practical reconstructions of image of the sun.
1961–1963	Oldendorf, Kuhl, Edwards, and Cormack	Applied reconstruction technique to medical problems.
1967	Hounsfield (England)	Worked on pattern recognition reconstruction techniques.
1967–1970	Hounsfield	Developed first clinically useful CT head scanner.
1971	Atkinson-Morley Hospital (England)	First clinically useful CT head scanner installed.
1972	Hounsfield and Ambrose	First paper on CT presented to British Institute of Radiology.
1973	Mayo Clinic (U.S.), Massachusetts General Hospital (U.S.)	First CT brain scanner installed.
1974	Ledley (U.S.)	Introduced whole-body CT scanner (ACTA scanner).

The growth of the CT has been dramatic. In the United States, for example, the number of scanners purchased in 1973 was about 30, while this number increased to about 100 in 1974, and to more than 300 whole-body and head scanners in 1975. The rate of growth continues to increase with time. Numerous manufacturers and research groups are actively involved in making further improvements and developments in the technology.

Although other workers investigated the idea of CT, it was Hounsfield who independently developed the first practical CT scanner. Therefore, he will be recognized as the man who opened up a whole new area of interest for radiologists, technologists, medical physicists, and other related scientists, just as Professor Roentgen did when he discovered x-rays.

Godfrey Hounsfield was born in 1919, in Nottinghamshire, England. After an outstanding performance at Magnus Grammar, he moved on to radar school at the Royal Air Force in Cranwell. There he undertook his formal education in electronics. After his student days he was appointed a lecturer at the same school. Following this, he attended Faraday House, where he studied electrical and mechanical engineering.

In 1951, he joined the staff at EMI, Limited, in London, where he began working on radar systems and later on computer technology. His research on computers led to the evolution of EMIDEC 1100, the first solid-state business computer in Britain.

In 1967, Hounsfield became interested in pattern recognition and reconstruction techniques using the computer. His research gave birth to the first clinically useful CT brain scanner. For this work, he received the equivalent of the Nobel Prize in Engineering, the McRobert Award, in 1972.

More recently (1979), Hounsfield shared the Nobel Prize in Physiology and Medicine with Allan MacLeod Cormack, a 55-year-old physics professor at Tufts University, Medford, Massachusetts, for work on CT.

Professor Cormack was born in Johannesburg, South Africa, in 1924. He attended the University of Capetown and then studied nuclear physics at Cambridge University. Later, he moved to the United States and did a sabbatical at Harvard University before joining the physics department at Tufts University. Professor Cormack developed solutions to mathematical problems involved in CT, which he has published in the *Journal of Applied Physics* in 1963 and 1964.

The clinical usefulness of CT is already well established in the diagnosis of diseases of the central nervous system. Disorders such as gliomas, metastases, intracranial lesions, aneurysms, infarctions, hemorrhage, atrophy, and so on, have been successfully detected by CT. In children, CT is useful in evaluating intracranial disorders such as hydrocephalus and neoplasms. At present, CT is more specific and more sensitive to the presence of primary and secondary neoplasms than is radionuclide scanning.

With the introduction of body scanners, CT of other parts of the body, such as the neck, thorax, abdomen, retroperitoneum, pelvis, and extremities, has, in some cases, produced definitive results. On the other hand, some controversies have arisen regarding the clinical efficacy of CT for other areas of the body. Despite these concerns, CT investigations of the body continue at a rapid rate.

CT is a noninvasive technique and does not cause discomfort to the patient or carry definite risks. It does not require hospitalization, as do cerebral angiography and pneumoencephalography. CT examinations can also reduce other problems related to patient management, such as postoperative care. For some examinations, however, the patient may receive an intravenous injection of iodine contrast medium prior to the scanning process. This enhances the contrast of certain internal structures. The contrast agent may cause some reaction in the patient, so the CT examination is not entirely hazard-free.

One of the major concerns in CT examination is the radiation dose, since x-radiation is damaging to most tissues. A fundamental objective in CT equipment design is to provide maximum information content with minimal radiation dose to the patient. Studies have indicated that the radiation dose in a CT brain scan is about equal to that received from a conventional skull x-ray examination requiring 6 to 10 films. Because the x-ray beam is well collimated, the amount of scattered radiation present during a CT scan is very small.

CT technology has already demonstrated how valuable physics, mathematics, and computer technology are to diagnostic radiology. A true understanding of CT will ultimately require at least a fundamental knowledge of computer technology and image reconstruction mathematics. At present, extensive research is being done on the physics and engineering aspects of CT; this research will ultimately be reflected in additional clinical benefits.

CT opens up a remarkable method of radiologic diagnosis. It is indeed a revolutionary evolution and a technological achievement. As time progresses, CT may become routine in most large-scale radiology departments. Therefore, every effort must be made to develop a fundamental understanding of the concepts underlying the principles of CT.

CHAPTER 1

FUNDAMENTALS OF THE COMPUTER

We are still in control, but the capabilities of computers are increasing at a fantastic rate while raw human intelligence is changing slowly, if at all. . . . In the 1990s, when the sixth generation appears, the compactness and reasoning power of an intelligence built out of silicon will begin to match that of the human brain.

ROBERT JASTROW,
Director, NASA Goddard Institute for Space Studies (1978)

The use of computers in society is growing rapidly. The introduction and evolution of computers have profoundly influenced the lives of each of us. Today, the computer is used in every facet of human activity, including business administration, government, military, education, science, medicine, architecture, engineering, communications, and research, to mention only a few. The use of the computer is advantageous because of its speed, accuracy, and capacity for storing information that can be easily retrieved.

The primary purpose of this chapter is to introduce some fundamental concepts and associated terminology of computer technology. It is imperative that those who work in the field of radiology gain a basic understanding of the computer, since it is beginning to receive widespread application in radiology.

DEFINITION OF A COMPUTER

The computer is a machine for solving problems. More specifically, a modern computer is a fast electronic computational machine that receives input data, processes the information by performing arithmetic or logical operations using a program stored in its memory, and generates output data that can be displayed on suitable output devices. In common usage this machine has come to be referred to as an "electronic computer" or simply "computer."

HISTORICAL NOTES

The history of computers and computing goes back about two hundred decades to the *abacus,* the first digital calculator, which was used for counting by sliding beads on wires (IBM, 1971).

No other counting machine found widespread use until 1642, when Blaise Pascal, the French mathematician, developed an *arithmetic machine.* Later, in 1694, Gottfried Wilhelm von Leibnitz completed a *calculating machine* for solving problems in multiplication and division. Following this, Jacquard in France developed an automatic loom in which the sequence of operations was based on coded information punched onto paper cards.

In 1822, Charles Babbage, a nineteenth-century English mathematician, developed a *difference engine,* a machine for calculating mathematical tables. Later he used the idea of punched-card coding to develop the *analytical engine,* a machine that solved mathematical problems automatically.

Around 1890, Dr. Herman Hollerith of the United States Census Office developed the first electrical tabulator (Fig. 1–1), based on a punched-card operation, which was used for the US Census of 1890 (IBM, 1971).

After this period, the development of computers progressed at a rapid rate. Since it is not the intent of this section to present a detailed account of computer history, only a summary of some important events will be listed here.

1937–1944	Howard Aiken at Harvard University developed the MARK 1 (automatic sequenced controlled calculator), a large electromechanical calculator.
1943–1946	At the University of Pennsylvania, Eckert and Mauchly developed the first electronic calculator, ENIAC (electronic numerical integrator and calculator).
1946–1952	The electronic computer EDVAC (electronic discrete variable automatic computer) was developed at the University of Pennsylvania by Eckert and Mauchly, while EDSAC was developed in England.
1951	UNIVAC (universal automatic computer) became the first commercially available computer.
1954	First computer used for business was fabricated and delivered to the General Electric Company (Davis, 1973; IBM, 1971).

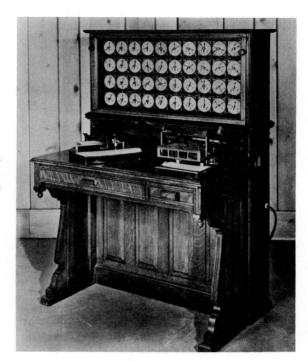

Figure 1–1. The first electrical tabulator developed by Dr. Herman Hollerith. (Courtesy of International Business Machines Corporation.)

In Figure 1–2, some other highlights in the development of the computer are shown.

Today, the computer has been developed to such a point that it is said to be in the fourth generation of its history (Couger and McFadden, 1977). The term *generation* is used to indicate that several significant changes have occurred throughout the development stages of the computer. In Table 1–1, four generations of computers and some characteristic features of each are given.

TABLE 1–1. SOME CHARACTERISTICS OF FOUR GENERATIONS OF COMPUTERS*

GENERATION	PRINCIPAL FEATURES
First	Vacuum tubes Data processing applications Expensive, relatively slow, unreliable Air-conditioned room needed
Second (introduced in 1959–1969)	Solid-state devices (transistors) Smaller, less heat production Less power requirements Reliable
Third (introduced in 1965)	Integrated circuits (including magnetic cores and semiconductors) Smaller still, greater speed and reliability
Fourth	Advanced storage system (miracle chips) Faster, smaller, less expensive than present-day computers

*After Couger, J. D., and McFadden, F. R.: A First Course in Data Processing. New York, John Wiley and Sons, Inc., 1977.

HIGHLIGHTS IN THE STORY OF THE CALCULATOR

From the abacus to the electronic computer, every improvement in calculating devices has come in answer to the need for faster and more efficient means of counting . . . releasing man from needless figuring and leaving him free to create.

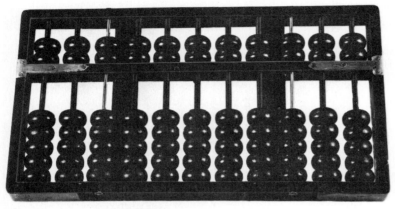

ABACUS

c. 1200   ("Suan-pan")   China

Calculator of antiquity which historians trace vaguely to Egypt, India, and Mesopotamia.

NAPIER'S RODS

1617   John Napier   Scotland

Mathematician and co-inventor of logarithms, Napier devised these computing rods to simplify multiplication. They were widely used during the seventeenth century.

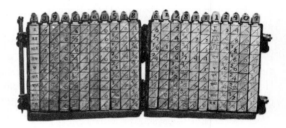

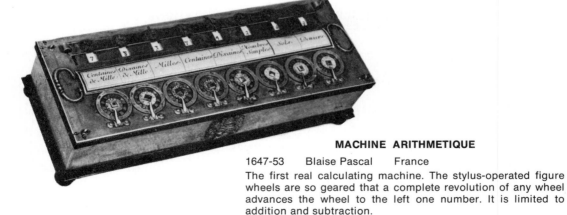

MACHINE ARITHMETIQUE

1647-53   Blaise Pascal   France

The first real calculating machine. The stylus-operated figure wheels are so geared that a complete revolution of any wheel advances the wheel to the left one number. It is limited to addition and subtraction.

Figure 1–2. Other highlights in the evolution of the computer. (Courtesy of International Business Machines Corporation.)

Illustration continued on opposite page

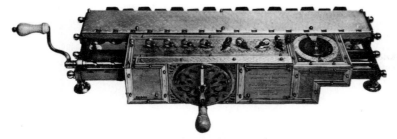

RECHENMASHINE

1673   Gottfried von Leibnitz   Germany

Designed to perform multiplication by rapidly repeated addition. The mechanism was not completely reliable, but the "stepped reckoner" principle which Leibnitz devised was used in the Thomas and other calculators.

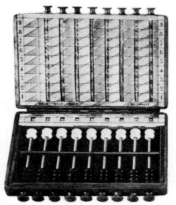

POCKET CALCULATOR

c. 1800   France

Combination of Chinese abacus and mechanized Napier's rods.

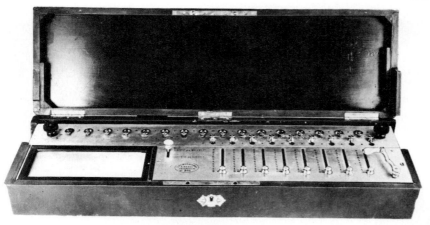

ARITHMOMETER

1820   Thomas de Colmar   France

This first commercially practical calculating machine used the Leibnitz "stepped reckoner" principle. Its manufacture was made possible by the new machine methods of the Industrial Revolution.

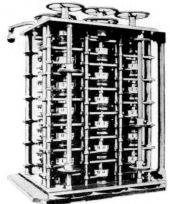

DIFFERENCE ENGINE

1823-33   Charles Babbage   England

The idea for a Difference Engine that would compute mathematical tables, such as logarithms, was first conceived by Babbage in 1812. After twenty years of labor, financial difficulties compelled him to stop work and the machine was never completed.

Illustration continued on following page

THE SCHEUTZ DIFFERENCE ENGINE

1834-53   Sweden

George Scheutz, aided by his son, was more
fortunate than Babbage, in that he completed
his Difference Engine. Patterning his machine
after the Babbage machine, he built several
models and finally perfected one which was
used to compute and print English Life Tables.

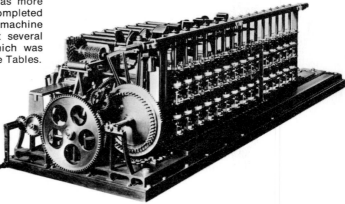

MACHINE A CALCULER

1889   Leon Bollee   France

The first calculating machine to perform
multiplication by the direct method and
not by repeated addition. It was never
produced commercially because of Bollee's greater interest in racing automo-
biles.

THE MILLIONAIRE

1892   Otto Steiger   Switzerland
The first successful multiplying machine. Using
tongued multiplication plates similar to those in-
vented by Bollee, the Millionaire was more compact
and enjoyed wide sale.

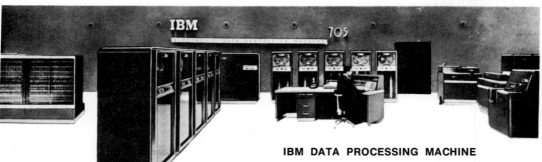

IBM DATA PROCESSING MACHINE

A giant electronic computer is not one, but a system of machines.
Its speed is measured in microseconds totaling many millions
of operations an hour. Its capacity taxes the imagination. Magnetic tapes, drums, and cores store vast
quantities of information which may be read and processed at speeds exceeding 58,000 characters per
second. Data output may be written at equally incredible speed on magnetic tapes or printed at a rate of
1000 lines a minute.

More recently, fifth-generation computers have become available, and these make use of special devices such as bubble memories and Josephson junctions (Jastrow, 1978).

Each new generation of computers has brought about a large increase in computing power (memory size and computing speed) along with significant decrease in cost. These two factors have caused the rapid growth of computer technology.

TYPES OF COMPUTERS

Computers are often classified according to *type, purpose,* and *size.* There are basically two types of computers, the *digital* computer (the most common type of computer) and the *analog* computer.

While digital computers solve problems by counting, analog computers measure continuous physical quantities. The signals are not digital but can have any value on a continuously variable scale (analog signals). The data that analog computers use vary continuously and generally involve physical quantities such as current, voltage, speed, pressure, displacement, and temperature.

The slide rule is a good example of an analog computer; here an analogy is made between length on the rule and the logarithm of a number. Another example is a computer in which a patient's heartbeat is converted into voltage. This voltage can be processed by electronic circuits and the results displayed on a CRT screen for analysis by a physician.

Different types of computers are referred to as *general-purpose* or *special-purpose* computers, depending on their use. Obviously, a special-purpose computer performs one or more specific functions, such as a reservation system of an airline or a tracker of missiles or satellites in space. A general-purpose computer, on the other hand, is designed to facilitate broader functions, such as solving science and engineering problems and data processing for business applications. The general-purpose computer performs this kind of processing by altering the stored program of instructions (O'Brien, 1979), unlike the "built-in" instructions of a special-purpose computer.

Today, computer sizes range from super, large, medium, small, and mini- to microcomputers, each having its own characteristics relating to input/output and storage capabilities, processing speeds, and cost.

A *minicomputer* is a small computer with a smaller memory, a slower processing speed, and fewer input/output capabilities (O'Brien, 1979) than small, medium, or large computers. The computer system used in CT is usually a minicomputer system.

A *microcomputer* is an extremely small computer such as one that has its circuitry on a "chip" or one that is about the size of a typewriter (O'Brien, 1979). It has the capabilities of a large computer, but with restricted storage and input/output capabilities and slower processing speeds. Because of this, the microcomputer has found common usage as a "personal computer" and is suitable for use in the home.

Small- and medium-scale computer systems are shown in Figures 1–3 and 1–13, respectively. A large-scale computer system is shown in the last picture of Figure 1–2.

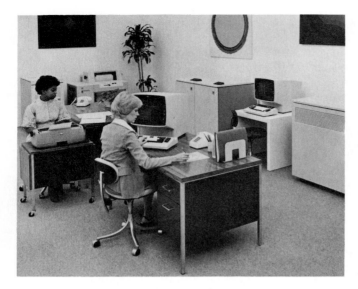

Figure 1–3. A small-scale computer system. (Courtesy of International Business Machines Corporation.)

THE DIGITAL COMPUTER

A digital computer solves problems by counting. It operates on digital (numerical) data through arithmetic or logical operations. The digital computer is widely used today, since it is easily adaptable to most data processing applications. Since the digital computer is used in radiologic applications, particularly computer tomography, the discussion that follows will apply mostly to digital computers. To understand how digital computers work, a review of the binary number system is in order.

NUMBER SYSTEMS

To understand the *binary number system,* one should first review the decimal number system.

The decimal number system (from the Latin *decem,* meaning "ten") has a *base* 10, in which the ten values are represented by 0, 1, 2, 3, 4, 5, 6, 7, 8, 9. Any number can be expressed as a sum of these digits, times a power of 10. For example,

$$(1 \times 10^0) + (2 \times 10^1) + (3 \times 10^2) = 321$$
$$= (1 \times 1) \quad + (2 \times 10) \quad + (3 \times 100) = 321$$
$$= \quad 1 \quad + \quad 20 \quad + \quad 300 \quad = 321$$

The number 321 is thus formed from units (1), tens (20), and hundreds (300). Hence any number in the decimal system can be written as units, tens, hundreds, thousands, tens of thousands, hundreds of thousands, millions, and so on. These powers of ten are indicated as:

$$1 \times 10^0 = 1$$
$$1 \times 10^1 = 10$$
$$1 \times 10^2 = 100$$
$$1 \times 10^3 = 1000$$
$$1 \times 10^4 = 10,000$$
$$1 \times 10^5 = 100,000$$
$$1 \times 10^6 = 1,000,000$$

The Binary Number System

In the binary number system, the *base* is 2 and the values are represented by 0 and 1. A binary number therefore is made up of only 0's and 1's. For example, the number 9 in the decimal system is 1001 in the binary system ($1 \times 2^3 + 0 \times 2^2 + 0 \times 2^1 + 1 \times 2^0$). Whereas each position value in the decimal system is *ten* times more than the position to its right, in the binary system each position value is *two* times more than the position to its right. Thus, the values, from right to left, are 1, 2, 4, 8, 16, 32, 64, 128, and so on.

The relationship between decimal and binary numbers is shown in the following chart.

Position Values	1000	100	10	1	8	4	2	1
				1	0	0	0	1
				2	0	0	1	0
				3	0	0	1	1
				4	0	1	0	0
				5	0	1	0	1
				6	0	1	1	0
				7	0	1	1	1
				8	1	0	0	0
				9	1	0	0	1
			1	0	1	0	1	0
			1	1	1	0	1	1
			1	2	1	1	0	0
			1	3	1	1	0	1
			1	4	1	1	1	0
			1	5	1	1	1	1

The columns are grouped under **DECIMAL** (Position Values 1000, 100, 10, 1) and **BINARY** (8, 4, 2, 1).

Other Number Systems

Binary numbers can become very long and hence may present time-consuming problems in reading them. One method of solving this problem is to use other number systems. Two such number systems are the octal and hexadecimal systems.

In the *octal system,* groups of three binary digits are represented by one octal digit. The *base* of the octal system is 8, in which the 8 digits are represented by 0, 1, 2, 3, 4, 5, 6, 7. For example, if the binary number is

$$010,110,100$$

then the octal number is 264; that is,
   a. Starting from the right of the binary number, group it into three's.
   b. Represent each group by an octal digit.
   c. 100 is thus 4.
   d. 110 is thus 6.
   e. 010 is thus 2.

Therefore, a string of 0's and 1's can easily be represented by the octal system, which is somewhat easier to deal with. The important point to remember is how the binary number system can be converted into the octal system.

The *hexadecimal system,* on the other hand, is a very efficient system for some computers. In this system 4 bits (binary digits) represent one hexadecimal digit, and the *base* is 16, in which the 16 digits are represented by 0, 1, 2, 3, 4, 5, 6, 7, 8, 9, 10, 11, 12, 13, 14, 15. In this case now, the first 10 digits are represented by 0, 1, 2, 3, 4, 5, 6, 7, 8, 9, while 10, 11, 12, 13, 14, and 15 are represented by the first six letters in the alphabet; that is A, B, C, D, E, and F, respectively. For example,

1101,1001 is the binary number.

The hexadecimal number is D9.

Solution:

a. Separate the binary digits into groups of 4 beginning from the right.
b. Figure out the hexadecimal equivalents; that is,

1001 is 9 and
1101 is 13

Since the first ten digits in the hexadecimal are represented by 0 through 9, then the hexadecimal number for the decimal equivalent 13 is D. Once again, the important point to remember here is that one hexadecimal number represents a four-digit binary number.

In the computer, the input data must be represented by certain codes. These codes could be one of several using the binary number system, such as a *4-bit code,* a *6-bit code,* and an *8-bit code.* In the 8-bit code, a group of 8 bits is called a *BYTE.* This is important for CT, since disk storage capacity (to be discussed later) is given in BYTES.

ELEMENTS IN A COMPUTER SYSTEM

Davies (1973) identifies five basic elements in a computer system. These are programs, procedures, personnel, software, and hardware. The *software* in a computer system represents all the instructions (programs, flow charts, etc.) prepared by people to allow the computer to solve problems. The *hardware* is the equipment portion of a computer. The workings of a computer can only be understood with a description of its equipment components. Hardware forms the functional units of the computer.

FUNCTIONAL UNITS OF A COMPUTER

In a contemporary computer system there are five functionally independent principal components. These are shown in Figure 1–4 and include:
a. Input devices
b. The central processing unit (CPU), which generally houses
   1. the arithmetic/logic unit (ALU)
   2. the memory unit
   3. the control unit
c. Output devices

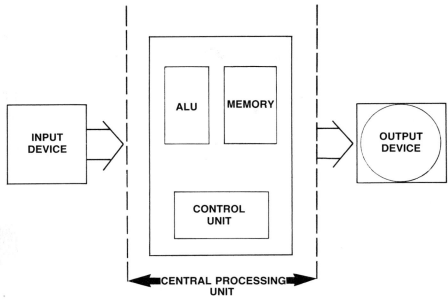

Figure 1–4. A typical method of organization of the functional units in a computer.

Input Devices

Input devices accept coded instructions. These instructions are sent to the CPU, where they are processed. The instructions can also be stored in the memory, for later use.

Input devices are units which "read" the data that are represented on the input medium, such as *paper tape* or *punched cards*. A card punch unit is shown in Figure 1–5. An input device is the *teletype,* which consists of a paper-

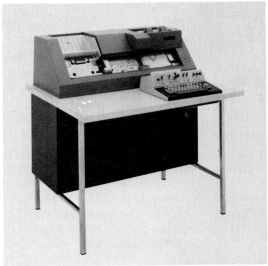

Figure 1–5. A keypunch machine. (Courtesy of International Business Machines Corporation.)

tape reader, a punch station, and a typewriter. The teletype is the most commonly used input device. Other input devices include *paper-tape readers* and *card readers,* which "read" the holes that are usually punched onto tapes and cards, respectively. Card readers are especially useful when large amounts of data are to be handled. Magnetic-ink readers and optical scanners are also examples of input devices.

Magnetic-ink readers are units that direct and read information printed with magnetic ink (iron oxide particles).

Optical scanners are units that read handwritten or typed information by scanning with a light and lens system and convert it to digital information.

Magnetic tape or disks can be used as a source of input. Here, a plastic tape or disk containing iron oxide particles is used to store the program by magnetizing the particles in a characteristic maneuver.

In summary, input devices are units that translate external data (such as holes on punched cards, keystrokes at a keyboard, magnetic tape, or magnetic disks) into internal binary representation for further manipulation.

Central Processing Unit (CPU)

The CPU is the heart of the computer system. As mentioned already, it consists of the arithmetic/logic unit, control circuits, and the memory unit. A CPU is shown in Figure 1–13.

Arithmetic/Logic Unit (ALU)

The ALU is used for computation purposes. Data are sent to the unit from the memory for arithmetic or logical operations to be performed on them. For example, the ALU can perform multiplication, addition, subtraction, and division. The appropriate computation is made, and the answer can be displayed immediately or stored in the memory. Logic operations (e.g., comparing numbers) can also be performed by the ALU.

Memory Unit

The memory unit stores information, such as data and programs, which the computer must locate when it is needed. For this purpose, the memory is divided into small regions called *locations*.

Information can be accessed from storage by stating where it is located; that is, by stating its *storage address*. This address is usually represented by a number. The computer identifies this number to read the stored information at that location, but does not remove it. However, when the computer stores new information, the "old" information is removed from its location.

There are two kinds of storage, primary and secondary. In *secondary storage,* devices such as magnetic disks, tapes, and drums are used. These are referred to as auxiliary memories, and they function to supplement the main memory. In CT, this kind of storage is commonly used.

Magnetic tape consists of a plastic base coated with iron oxide or other metallic particles. The tape is threaded from a supply reel to pass by a special device called a read-write head, and onto a take-up reel, as shown in Figure 1–6A.

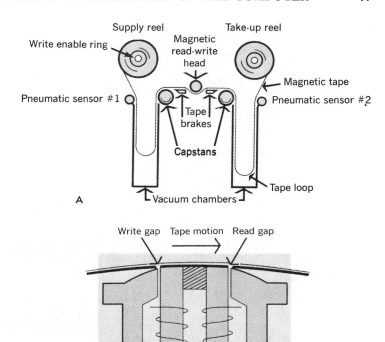

Figure 1–6. Threading of magnetic tape from reel to reel *(A)* to pass by the read-write head *(B)*. (From Davis, G.B.: Computer Data Processing, 2nd Ed. New York, McGraw-Hill Book Company, 1973. Reproduced by permission.)

The *read-write head* is made of an iron core with a small gap or gaps and a wire wrapped around the core (Fig. 1–6*B*). In recording (writing) information on the tape, a varying electrical signal (passing through the wire) produces a varying magnetic field that magnetizes the iron particles in the tape and is thus recorded. The direction of the magnetization of the tape represents 0's and 1's (binary numbers). In playback (reading), the magnetized iron particles, when passed over the magnetic tape head, produce electrical signals which then go on to other devices such as a TV or speaker. Figure 1–7 shows the magnetic tape unit.

A *magnetic disk* resembles a phonograph record. It is a metal disk with a coating of magnetic material (ferrous oxide) on both sides. The disk has concentric tracks (rings) and preshaped sectors (Fig. 1–8). In locating information on the disk, both the track and the sector are identified by a special device, the read-write head. Figure 1–9 shows a disk storage unit.

The *floppy disk,* also referred to as a diskette, is a modification of the magnetic disk. It is small, thin, and flexible — hence the term *floppy*. The diskette shown in Figure 1–10 is used in CT to store individual patient images.

Finally, a *magnetic drum* is a geometric cylinder, the surface of which is coated with magnetic material and which rotates during storage and retrieval of data. The location of the data is identified by a set of stationary read-write heads located near the surface of the drum.

For secondary storage using magnetic tape, the information put on the tape is not addressable; therefore, to find any specific information, the tape must be searched until such information is located. The device used to acquire access to such information is called a *sequential access device.*

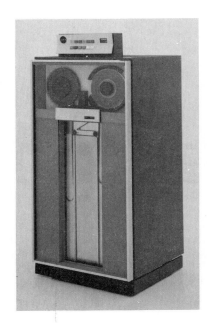

Figure 1–7.   A magnetic tape unit. (Courtesy of International Business Machines Corporation.)

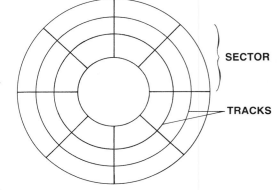

Figure 1–8.   Schematic of magnetic disk showing tracks and sectors.

SECTOR

TRACKS

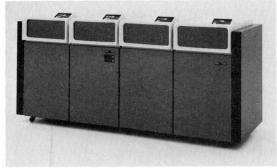

Figure 1–9.   A disk storage unit. (Courtesy of International Business Machines Corporation.)

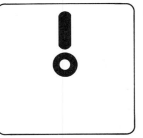

Figure 1–10.   A diagrammatic representation of a floppy disk. The disk is used in CT as a secondary storage device.

For secondary storage using magnetic disks, the information stored on the disk can be found very quickly, since *direct access devices* are used to locate the information. Such devices have addressable storage locations.

Information can be fetched much more rapidly from *primary storage,* i.e., magnetic cores (Fig. 1–11) (core memories) and more recently semiconductor chips (semiconductor memories). In this kind of storage the information can be accessed by stating its address. Such *semiconductor memories* or *integrated circuits,* as they are often referred to, are used in present-day computers. A semiconductor is a solid crystalline substance whose properties of electrical conductivity fall between those of a conductor and those of an insulator. Two examples of semiconductor materials are germanium and silicon.

Semiconductor memories consist of transistors or diodes that have two states, thus allowing current to be either "on" or "off." Semiconductor chips are used today in computers, since they are faster and smaller than magnetic cores and thus have larger storage capacities for their size. The semiconductor chip shown in Figure 1–12 can hold up to 64,000 bits of information equivalent to 1,000 eight-letter words.

The memory *storage capacity* is described according to the number of addressable locations. It is indicated usually by the letter K (kilo), which is

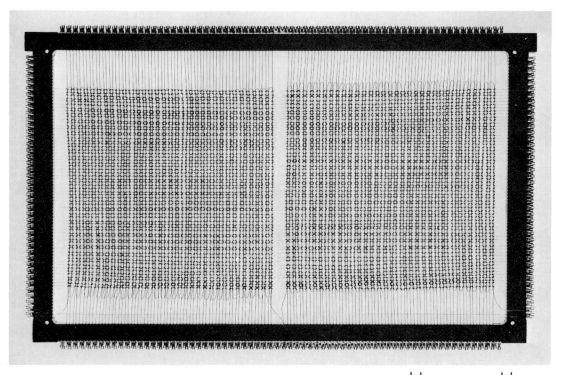

A

Figure 1–11. *A,* An array of magnetic cores used in older computers (third generation) for primary storage. These cores are tiny doughnut-shaped ferrite rings fitted around intersecting wires that carry current. The current produces magnetization in the core in clockwise or counterclockwise directions to represent 0's and 1's. (Courtesy of International Business Machines Corporation.) *B,* A schematic of a single magnetic core.

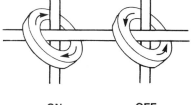

B   ON   OFF

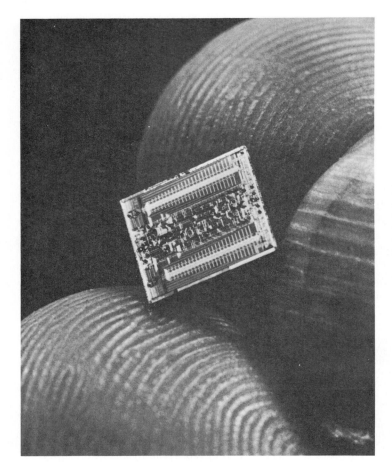

Figure 1–12. A semiconductor memory chip. This 64,000-bit chip was developed at IBM's General Technology Division Laboratory in Vermont. (Courtesy of International Business Machines Corporation.)

used to represent thousands. Thus a 64K memory has about 64,000 positions or locations. Computers in CT have storage capacities that vary; some have memories of 32K, 64K, 96K, 128K, etc.

Control Unit

The operation of the units described so far is coordinated by the control unit. It directs all other units by using programs that are stored in the memory and sends data to the arithmetic unit to be processed, after which it sends the information back to the memory for storage or to an appropriate output device for display. For example, a line printer (an output device) will respond (i.e., print a line) only when instructed by the control unit.

The Computer Console

The console of a computer usually consists of a control panel coupled to either a typewriter (Fig. 1–13) and/or a CRT device with a keyboard. The numerous buttons and switches on the control panel of the computer console plus the keyboard on the typewriter or CRT device allow the operator to "communicate" with the CPU by entering data or instructions.

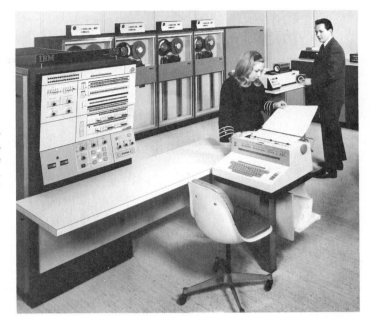

Figure 1–13. A computer console with typewriter. The unit showing the console is also the CPU. (Courtesy of International Business Machines Corporation.)

The series of lights on the console serves to indicate how the system is functioning and also identifies problems in any component in the computer.

Output Devices

These devices are used to display the results of a computation so that they can be easily interpreted by the people operating them. Examples of output devices include a *high-speed printer* (such as the one shown in Figure 1–14), *card punch, paper-tape punch,* and the *cathode ray tube* (CRT) display device, which is very commonly used (Fig. 1–15). The unit in Figure 1–15 is also an example of a device that can be used as both an input and an output device. In this case, the keyboard represents the input, and the output is displayed on the CRT screen.

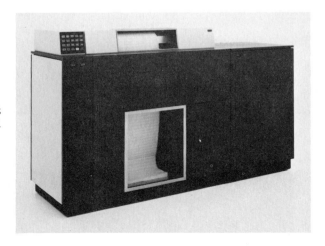

Figure 1–14. A high-speed output printer. (Courtesy of International Business Machines Corporation.)

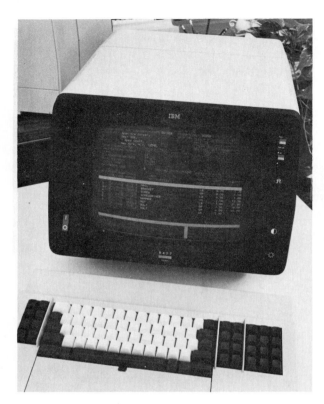

Figure 1–15. A cathode ray tube (CRT) output display device. The design model shown here can display up to 3440 characters on its tilted antireflective screen. (Courtesy of International Business Machines Corporation.)

PROGRAMMING

The operation of a computer is directed by a complete set of directions called a *program*. It specifies the steps necessary to solve a problem.

The program is prepared by people who are referred to as *programmers*.

Once a program is prepared, it must be translated into some form usable by both the computer and the programmer. For this purpose, a number of codes have been developed and are now used today. These codes include machine language (binary representation as stored in the memory) and higher-level languages such as COBOL (Common Business-Oriented Language) and FORTRAN (Formula Translator), which is suitable for use in science and engineering and research. Other high-level languages are BASIC (Beginners All-purpose Symbolic Instruction Code), ALGOL (Algorithmic Language), APL (A Programming Language), and PL/1 (Programming Language, Version 1), which are all used in stating formulas and solving mathematical problems.

In preparing a program, the programmer must set up a scheme of action to be used by the computer in solving the problem. The scheme is called a *flowchart*. In planning the flowchart, a number of flowchart symbols are used to indicate the sequence of operations that must be carried out. Figure 1–16 illustrates some common flowchart symbols used in computer programming.

The programming used in CT to direct the mathematical operations in producing the CT image is extremely complex and hence will not be discussed in this text.

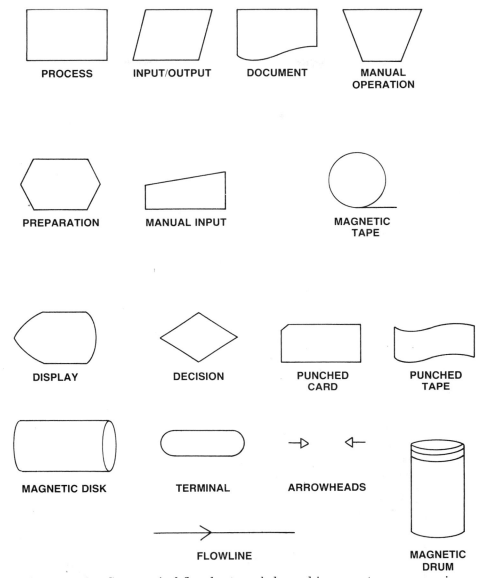

Figure 1–16. Some typical flowchart symbols used in computer programming.

HOW A COMPUTER WORKS — AN OVERVIEW

The workings of a computer can be simplified in the following way. First, the data to be processed must be represented in some way. Coding systems are used to represent the data. For example, the binary number system, together with other number systems (already described) are used by digital computers.

The data are sent to the computer through the input unit. They can also be stored in the memory for later use.

Steps   Comments

1 **Analysis of a problem**   Proposed report   Collect information and decide what information is needed, frequency of processing, etc.

2 Design of a system to provide the information   **Plan the system of processing using a system flowchart plus layouts (diagrams) of reports, documents, records, files, etc.**

3 Planning the computer logic   Plan the program logic using a program flowchart and other methods of describing a program.

4 Program preparation   READ DATA. ADD A AND B GIVING C.   Write the program of instructions and debug it to remove all textual or logical errors. Translate it into machine language. Prepare documentation.

5 Input data preparation   Document   Key-punching   Punched card   Prepare input data by collecting or transcribing data into machine-readable form such as punched cards.

6 Running of program   Program   Input   Computer   Output   Put program into computer memory. Computer program reads data, processes it, and outputs the result.

7 Use of the output   Report

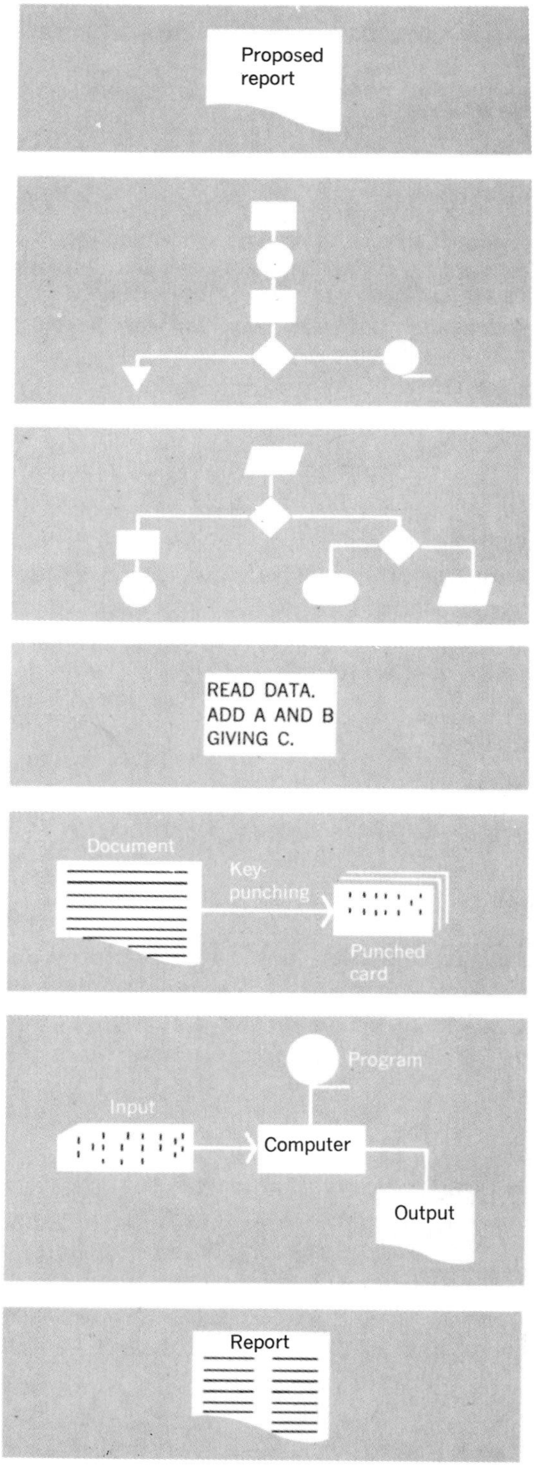

Figure 1–17. Steps in using the computer for information processing. (From Davis, G.B.: Computer Data Processing, 2nd Ed. New York, McGraw-Hill Book Company, 1973. Reproduced by permission.)

When a computation is to be made, the data are then taken from the memory and are sent to the ALU for processing. The results of the computation are sent to an appropriate output device for display or back to the memory for storage.

The function of all units of the computer is under the direct influence of the control unit.

Finally, the sequence of events in using the computer for processing information is shown in Figure 1–17.

This summary is only a superficial sketch of the workings of a computer. To fully understand a computer system, one must take a course in computer science. Such courses are becoming commonplace in almost every post-secondary institution in North America.

COMPUTER APPLICATIONS IN RADIOLOGY

Computer applications continue to increase at a rapid rate. Already computer applications in radiology are beginning to receive widespread attention.

It all began in 1955 when K. C. Tsien used the computer to calculate radiation dose distributions in cancer patients. Since his approach was mathematical, the use of the computer proved fruitful.

Today, computer applications in radiology (Lodwick, 1975) include:
  a. Dosimetry for radiation treatment planning.
  b. Radiologic reporting.
  c. Radiologic accounting and billing.
  d. Imaging.

The Need for Computer Applications in Radiology

Since radiology is a complex field and involves several processes in the production of the final end-product, the radiograph, the use of the computer is beneficial for several reasons. James et al. (1975) point out that the computer serves "to reduce human error, improve work efficiency, improve diagnostic effectiveness and eliminate delays in report transmission."

Radiologic Information Systems Application

The scientific literature is filled with reports of this kind of application. Several of these include works by Brolin (1972), Du Boulay and Price (1968), Pendergrass et al. (1969), Uber et al. (1968), Vogt et al. (1969), and Wheeler and Simborg (1975), to mention only a few. Mani and Jones (1973) have classified these applications into three groups based on the processing mode used by the computer.

It is not within the scope of this section to describe these applications; however, the interested reader should refer to the work of Mani and Jones (1973).

IMAGING APPLICATIONS

The purpose of imaging applications is primarily to improve the quality of radiologic diagnosis. These applications include:

a. Computer aided diagnosis (CAD).
b. Automated image analysis (AIA).
c. Computed tomography (CT).

Computed tomography is the most widely used. The other two applications (AIA and CAD) will not be discussed here, since they involve rigorous mathematical techniques. However, those who are interested in such applications should refer to the work of Lodwick (1975) and a review paper by Seeram (1976).

Undoubtedly, applications of the computer in radiology will continue to be made. The results of these applications have indicated that the efforts are very much worthwhile, whatever trend continues.

DIGITAL IMAGE PROCESSING — AN OVERVIEW

The fundamental basis of CT lies in the domain of *digital image processing*. An understanding of the elements of digital image processing is therefore essential for a clear comprehension of CT and, more importantly, of the role of the computer in reconstructing an image.

Digital image processing involves the conversion of a picture into numerical data (digitization) using a computer to process the information. First, the image is *scanned*. This means that the image is divided into small areas referred to as *picture elements*, or *pixels* for short. The results of the scanning show a grid on the image which consists of rows and columns.

The second step involves a *sampling* process in which the brightness or gray level is measured at each pixel location. This is done by using a number of devices such as a photomultiplier tube, which converts light into an electrical signal (Castleman, 1979).

In the third step, the data from sampling are *quantized*. In quantization, an integer (0 and positive and negative numbers) is used to represent the measured values obtained as a result of sampling (Castleman, 1979). The integer is referred to as the *gray level*. The final result of quantization of the entire image is an array of integers, with each pixel having a specific row or line number and a column or sample number (addresses) together with a digital integer (gray level) value (Castleman, 1979).

The digital data (obtained from the steps of scanning, sampling, and quantization) that are generated by the image digitizer are sent to the computer for processing. In this system, three elements are important, those of input, processing, and output. The input data are fed into the computer. Upon receiving instructions from the job control unit, the computer uses programs from the program library to process the information having read the input image line by line.

In processing, suitable programs are used to generate the output image pixel by pixel (Castleman, 1979). This image is then stored and/or fed into a digital display unit. In displaying the output image, the integers (gray levels) of individual pixels are utilized in establishing dark and light regions on the screen. It is interesting to note here that the human eye can perceive only about 40 shades of gray (Castleman, 1979).

HANDLING DIGITAL DATA IN CT

In CT, the general series of steps in digitizing an image is followed. The object is sampled through a specific scanning sequence (specific motions of the x-ray tube and detectors). The radiation beams used (primary and transmitted) are detected by suitable detectors, which convert x-ray photons into electrical signals. These signals are then quantized to generate integers proportional to the electrical energy, and hence the intensity of the radiation beam. Finally, an output device (magnetic tape or disk) stores the data, later to be used by the computer, which reconstructs from the data an image of the object that is scanned.

Figures 1–18 and 1–19 illustrate how digital data are transferred to the computer and stored for two types of CT systems. The motion of the x-ray tube and detectors and other important parameters will be explained in greater detail in Chapter 2.

ANALOG-TO-DIGITAL CONVERSION

Analog signals are those that vary continuously with time (e.g., voltage). These signals are useful in certain situations such as providing meter readings or displaying wave forms on an oscilloscope, but they cannot be used by a digital computer. Analog signals must therefore be converted into digital form before the computer can process them. The device used to perform this function is the *analog-to-digital (A/D) converter.*

The A/D converter consists of a frequency generator and comparator, often referred to as a "clock," which is made up of solid-state electronic circuits designed to change the analog signal into a digital number.

Consider Figure 1–20. The circuits of the "clock" are designed so that they will measure very small portions of the analog signal (voltage) and assign a

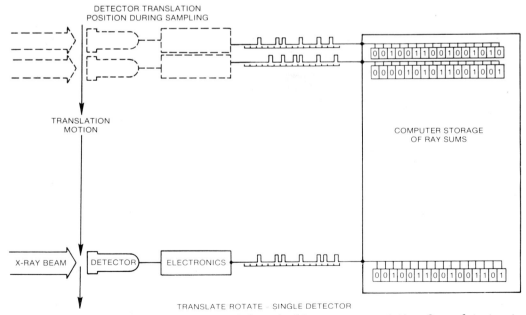

Figure 1–18. Transfer and storage of data in binary representation from detector to computer in a CT scanner with a single detector. (Courtesy of General Electric, Medical Systems Division, 1978.)

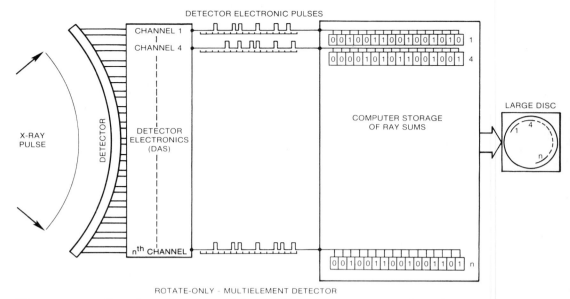

CHANNEL 1

CHANNEL 4

X-RAY PULSE

DETECTOR

DETECTOR ELECTRONICS (DAS)

nth CHANNEL

COMPUTER STORAGE OF RAY SUMS

LARGE DISC

ROTATE-ONLY - MULTIELEMENT DETECTOR

Figure 1–19. Transfer and storage of data in binary representation from detectors to computer in a CT scanner with multiple detectors. (Courtesy of General Electric, Medical Systems Division, 1978.)

numerical value to these portions. The output will then be in digital form. In the same figure, at the point where the value is shown to be 10 volts, the output digital binary value corresponding to that point will be 001010, which is the binary representation for 10. The computer can now use this information in the computational process.

DIGITAL-TO-ANALOG CONVERSION

When the digital data are processed by the computer, the results must be displayed in some form that people can understand. They can either be displayed as a "numerical" picture (digital) or be displayed on a CRT screen. In the latter case, the digital data must be converted to an analog signal. For this conversion the *digital-to-analog (D/A) converter* is used. The converter consists of solid-state electronics that will generate an output voltage proportional to the input digital number.

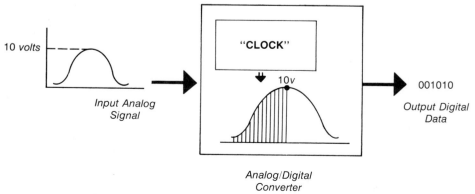

10 volts

"CLOCK"

10v

001010

Input Analog Signal

Output Digital Data

Analog/Digital Converter

Figure 1–20. Analog/digital conversion. See text for explanation.

CT / 1

SUMMARY/REFERENCES/BIBLIOGRAPHY/REVIEW QUESTIONS

Summary

1. This chapter presents an overview of the computer with respect to what it is and how it works. It also describes a few essential basic elements of digital image processing, since they form the basis for CT.

2. A computer is an electronic machine for solving problems by using arithmetic and logical operations through a set of instructions stored in its memory. The flow pattern for computer processing involves input, processing, and output.

3. Historical events in the development of the computer, beginning with the abacus and terminating with fourth-generation computers, are presented. Essential components characteristic of each generation, such as vacuum tubes, solid-state devices, and integrated circuits are given in table form.

4. A digital computer solves problems by counting, through operations on numerical (digital) data.

5. Data representation in the digital computer is based on the binary number, since devices in the computer work on two states, that is, "on" and "off." This is one coding system used in computers. Other coding systems (e.g., octal and hexadecimal) are also described.

6. The elements of a computer system include hardware, software, programs, procedures, and personnel. Only two of these were explained at this point in the chapter. Software refers to the programs that direct the operation of the computer.

7. The hardware components form the functional units of the computer. These include input devices, the arithmetic/logic unit, the memory, the control unit, and output devices.

8. Input devices feed data into the computer. These include teletypewriters, punched-card readers, and paper-tape readers.
    The ALU, the memory, and the control unit are all housed in the central processing unit.

9. The data are processed by the ALU by performing calculations on them given by the program.

10. The data may be stored in the memory, which contains programs for processing the data. Primary storage involves the use of magnetic cores and more recently semiconductor memories. In secondary storage, devices such as magnetic drums, magnetic disks, floppy disks, and magnetic tape are used.

11. The memory storage capacity is expressed according to the number of addressable locations and is usually indicated by the letter K, which is used to represent thousands.

12. The control unit regulates all activities within the computer, through interpretations of the program stored in the memory.

13. The computer console consists of a control panel and a typewriter or a CRT display device with a keyboard.

14.   Output devices are used to display the results of a computation. These may be line printers, cathode ray tubes, etc.

15.   A computer program is a set of instructions that direct the operation of the computer. In preparing a program, the programmer uses a flowchart to indicate the sequence of operations that must be carried out for optimum processing.

16.   Other computers that were described include the analog, general-purpose, special-purpose, and mini- and microcomputers. Analog computers solve problems by operating on continuous data.

17.   Computer applications in radiology include radiologic information systems, imaging, and dosimetry calculations for therapy.
Radiologic information systems include billing, accounting, clerical, and reporting. These were not discussed, since they are not within the scope of this book. Imaging applications include computer-aided diagnosis, automated image analysis, and computed tomography.

18.   Since the fundamental basis of CT relates to digital image processing, several elements were presented as an overview to a clearer comprehension of CT.
In digital image processing, those elements involve scanning the image, sampling, and quantization. In scanning, the image is divided into picture elements called pixels. Sampling involves a measurement of the brightness at each pixel location. Quantization is used to assign integers to the measured values obtained as a result of sampling. The integer is referred to as the gray level.

19.   In CT, similar steps in digitizing an image are used, except in this case the scanning involves specific motions of the x-ray tube and detectors.

20.   Since the computer can work only with binary data, the analog/digital converter was described. This converter is a device which changes an analog signal (voltage) to digital data, which the computer can then use. The digital/analog converter, on the other hand, changes digital data to analog signals which are used to display the results of processing input digital data.

References

Barnhard, H. J., and Cockray, K. T.: Computerized operation in the diagnostic radiology department. Am. J. Roentgenol., *109*:628–635, 1970.

Brolin, I.: MEDELA. An electronic data processing system for radiological reporting. Radiology, *103*:249–255, 1970.

Castleman, K. R.: Digital Image Processing. Englewood Cliffs, N.J., Prentice-Hall, Inc., 1979.

Couger, J. D., and McFadden, F. R.: A First Course in Data Processing. New York, John Wiley and Sons, Inc., 1977.

Coulson, J. M., and Richardson, J. F.: Computers and methods for computation. *In* Richardson, J. F., and Peacock D. G. (Eds.): Chemical Engineering, Vol. III. Elmsford, N.Y., Pergamon Press, 1971.

Davis, G. B.: Computer Data Processing, 2nd Ed. New York, McGraw-Hill Book Company, 1973.

DuBoulay, G. H., and Price, V. E.: The diagnosis of intracranial tumors assisted by computer. Br. J. Radiol., *41*:762–781, 1968.

Handel, S.: The Electronic Revolution. New York, Penguin Books, 1967.

Hollingdale, S. H., and Tootill, G. C.: Electronic Computers. New York, Penguin Books, 1971.

IBM: More About Computers. New York, International Business Machines Corporation, 1971.

James, W. B., Fulton, A., and Reekie, D.: Initial experience with a small dedicated computer system in a diagnostic x-ray department. Clin. Radiol., *26*:555–560, 1975.

Jastrow, R.: Toward an intelligence beyond man's. Time, Feb. 20, 1978.

Lodwick, G. S.: The application of computers in diagnostic radiology. *In* Baker, D. H., et al. (Eds.): Current Problems in Radiology, *5*:1–56, 1975.

Mani, R. L., and Jones, M. D.: MSF: A computer-assisted radiologic reporting system. Conceptual framework. Radiology, *108*:587–596, 1973.

O'Brien, J.: Computers in Business Management — An Introduction. Chicago, Richard D. Irwin, Inc., 1979.

Pendergrass, H. P., Greenes, R. A., Barnett, G. O., et al.: An on-line computer facility for systematized input of radiology reports. Radiology, *92*:709–713, 1969.

Seeram, E.: The computer and its applications in diagnostic radiology. Can. J. Radiog. Radiother. Nucl. Med., 7:238–246, 1976.

Stone, H. S.: Introduction to Data Structures and Computer Organization. New York, McGraw-Hill Book Company, 1972.

Templeton, A. W., et al.: RADIATE — up-dated and redesigned for multiple cathode ray tube terminals. Radiology, *92*:30–36, 1969.

Tsien, K. C.: The application of automatic computing machines to radiation treatment planning. Br. J. Radiol., *28*:432–435, 1955.

Uber, G. T., et al.: System for recording neuroradiologic diagnosis in a computer. Radiology, *91*:241–247, 1968.

Vogt, F. B., et al.: Use of a digital computer in measurement of roentgenographic bone density. Am. J. Roentgenol., *105*:870–876, 1969.

Wheeler, P. S., Simborg, D. W., and Gitlin, J. N.: The Johns Hopkins radiology reporting system. Radiology, *119*:315–319, 1976.

Bibliography

IBM: More About Computers. New York, International Business Machines Corporation, 1971.

Jastrow, R.: Toward an intelligence beyond man's. Time, Feb. 20, 1978.

Seeram, E.: The computer and its applications in diagnostic radiography. Can. J. Radiog. Radiother. Nucl. Med., 7:238–246, 1976.

Wheeler, P. S., Simborg, D. W., and Gitlin, J. N.: The Johns Hopkins radiology reporting system. Radiology, *119*:315–319, 1976.

Review Questions

1. Computer processing involves:
   - (a) Input, output, and processing.
   - (b) Input, processing, and output.
   - (c) Input, programming, and results.
   - (d) Programming, output, and processing.

2. Which of the following is indicative of first-generation computers?
   - (a) Vacuum tubes
   - (b) Integrated circuits
   - (c) Solid-state devices
   - (d) Josephson junctions

3. Transistors are used in which of the following?
   - (a) First-generation computers
   - (b) Second-generation computers
   - (c) Third-generation computers
   - (d) Fourth-generation computers

4. The binary representation 11001 is equivalent to the decimal number:
   - (a) 25
   - (b) 24
   - (c) 6
   - (d) 31

5. The decimal number 18 is equivalent to the binary number:
   - (a) 0001
   - (b) 10001
   - (c) 10010
   - (d) 11010

6. Which of the following is not part of the CPU?
   - (a) The ALU
   - (b) Memory unit
   - (c) Control unit
   - (d) Cathode ray tube

7. Which is an example of computer software?
   (a) The line printer
   (b) The computer program
   (c) The cathode ray tube
   (d) The control unit

8. Which of the following coordinates the activities of the computer?
   (a) The memory
   (b) The output device
   (c) The control unit
   (d) Input devices

9. Which of the following is a component of primary storage?
   (a) Magnetic drum
   (b) Magnetic tape
   (c) Magnetic disk
   (d) Magnetic cores

10. A flowchart is:
    (a) An illustration using specific symbols showing the sequence of operations in computer data processing.
    (b) A language used in business data processing.
    (c) A series of symbols shown on a template.
    (d) Another name for data processing.

11. Which of the following describes the storage capacity of the computer?
    (a) The number of secondary storage devices used in the computer system.
    (b) The number of input/output devices.
    (c) The number of addressable locations.
    (d) A group of binary digits.

12. A minicomputer:
    (a) Has a large memory capability.
    (b) Has a large number of input/output devices.
    (c) Is the size of a typewriter.
    (d) Has fewer input/output capabilities.

13. Which of the following is *not* an x-ray imaging application of the computer?
    (a) Computer-aided diagnosis.
    (b) Automated image analysis.
    (c) Computed tomography.
    (d) Radiologic information systems.

14. A pixel, as used in digital image processing, is:
    (a) A picture element.
    (b) A device that converts electricity into digits.
    (c) An integer.
    (d) A shade of gray.

15. An A/D converter:
    (a) Is an input device.
    (b) Converts binary digits into voltage.
    (c) Converts binary digits into a graphic display.
    (d) Converts voltage into binary representation.

16. The following is the basic flow pattern in digital image processing:
    (a) Scanning, sampling, and quantization.
    (b) Scanning, quantization, and sampling.
    (c) Sampling, scanning, and quantization.
    (d) Quantization, scanning, and sampling.

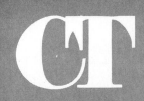

CHAPTER 2

PRINCIPLES OF COMPUTED TOMOGRAPHY

As in most radiologic procedures, the variable forming the CT image is the difference in x-ray attentuation properties of the various tissues.

M. M. TER-POGOSSIAN (1976)

Computed tomography (CT) is probably the most significant development in the history of medical imaging since the discovery of x-rays in 1895. The information presented in a CT image is different from that in a conventional radiographic image. The most conspicuous difference is that CT shows cross-sectional views of patient anatomy (Fig. 2–1). However, there are other important and significant differences in CT imaging.

In presenting the principles of CT, a review of conventional tomography and the limitations of radiography is helpful in understanding the value of the CT image.

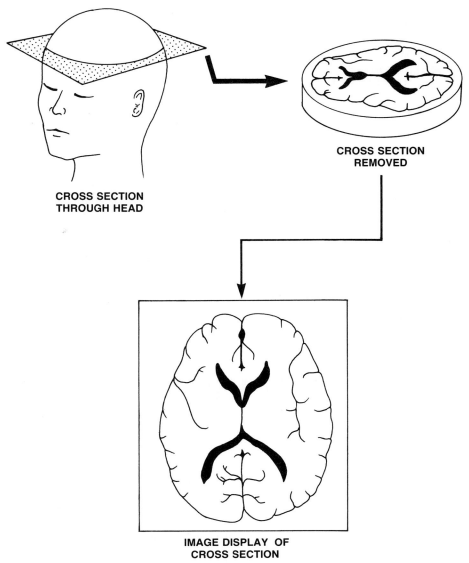

**CROSS SECTION
REMOVED**

**CROSS SECTION
THROUGH HEAD**

**IMAGE DISPLAY OF
CROSS SECTION**

Figure 2–1.   Schematic of cross-sectional imaging by computed tomography.

LIMITATIONS OF CONVENTIONAL RADIOGRAPHY AND TOMOGRAPHY

Limitations of Conventional Radiography

The major shortcoming of radiography is that of superimposition of all structures on the film (Fig. 2–2), which makes it difficult and sometimes impossible to distinguish a particular detail. This is especially true when the structures differ only slightly in density, as is often the case with some tumors and the tissues in which they are located. Although multiple views can be taken to localize a structure, the problem of superimposition in radiography still persists.

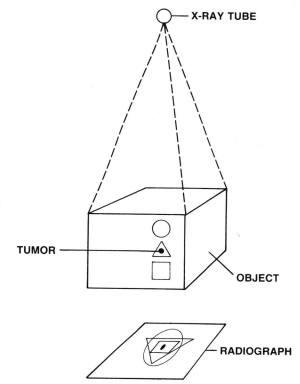

Figure 2–2. A major shortcoming of radiography. Superimposition of all structures on the radiograph makes it very difficult to discriminate whether the tumor is in the circle, triangle, or square.

Another limitation in radiography is that the procedure is qualitative and not quantitative. This simply means that a radiograph "does not distinguish between a homogeneous object of non-uniform thickness and a uniformly thick object of varying composition" (Marshall, 1976). This limitation is shown in Figure 2–3.

Limitations of Conventional Tomography

The problem of superimposition common to radiography can be overcome somewhat by conventional tomography (Bocage, 1974; Vallebona, 1931). Figure 2–4 shows the most common method of geometric tomography. By simultaneously moving the x-ray tube and film in opposite directions, unwanted sections can be blurred out while the desired layer is kept "in focus."

The immediate objective in tomography is to eliminate the layers outside the focused section (focal plane). However, this is quite difficult to achieve, and under no circumstances can all unwanted planes be blurred out.

Tomography then, poses several limitations, including (a) image blurring that persists and cannot be completely removed, (b) degradation of contrast due to the presence of scattered radiation, and (c) other limitations due to x-ray film/screen combinations (McCullough, 1976).

Both radiography and tomography fail to demonstrate adequately slight differences in subject contrast characteristic of soft tissues of the body (McCullough, 1976). For example, attenuation coefficients for human fat, water, human cerebrospinal fluid, human plasma, monkey pancreas, monkey white matter, monkey gray matter, monkey liver, monkey muscle, and human

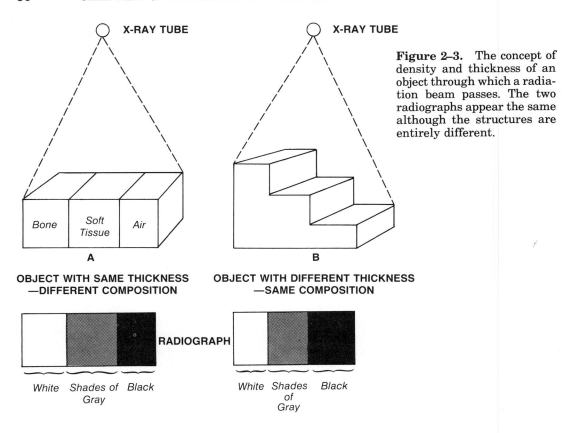

Figure 2–3. The concept of density and thickness of an object through which a radiation beam passes. The two radiographs appear the same although the structures are entirely different.

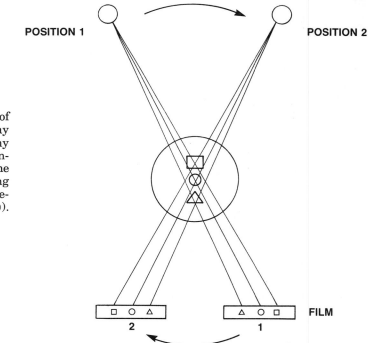

Figure 2–4. Basic principles of geometric tomography. The x-ray tube and film move in synchrony and in opposite directions to ensure that a desired section of the patient (○) is imaged by blurring out structures above (□) and below (△) the plane of interest (○).

red cells are 0.194, 0.222, 0.227, 0.227, 0.230, 0.230, 0.235, 0.236, 0.238, and 0.247, respectively (Ter-Pogossian et al., 1974).

Today these limitations are overcome by CT, which has been developed so that it can image tissue contrast with excellent discrimination.

DEFINITION OF CT

CT is a new type of cross-sectional tomographic imaging in which all unwanted planes or layers of a body are completely eliminated using mathematical techniques. The goal of CT is to detect radiation that has passed through a body (e.g., patient) at multiple angles, and with the aid of a computer, to reconstruct a cross section of absorption values for that body section. The computer is used to store the data (x-ray transmission values) and reconstruct an image from these data.

Many terms have been used to describe this technique. CT is thus synonymous with computerized transverse axial tomography (CTAT), computer-assisted tomography or computerized axial tomography (CAT), computerized tomography (CT), reconstructive tomography (RT), and computerized transaxial transmission reconstructive tomography (CTT). The term *computed tomography* has recently been established by *Radiology* and the *American Journal of Roentgenology,* and has received widespread acceptance in the radiologic community. Throughout the remainder of this text, the term *computed tomography* and its abbreviation CT will be used.

In summary, CT involves reconstructions from x-ray transmission measurements through the patient. The information is processed by a computer, which uses mathematical techniques to generate a picture of the internal structures in cross section.

PHYSICAL BASIS

Data Acquisition

The main objective in CT is to produce a series of images using a "tomographic method" (Fig. 2–5), in which each of the images in the lower row is derived from a specific tomographic "cut" (Hounsfield, 1973). The images are sharp and free of any superimposition from both overlying and underlying structures.

The CT image depends upon several steps illustrated in Figure 2–6. These steps form the essential elements of any CT system:

1. The x-ray tube and detector traverse (scan) the object. A number of discrete readings are made during each scan. This number varies from 160 to 320 or more for different scanners.

2. The radiation beam passes through the object and is attenuated. The transmitted photons are detected by suitable detectors placed behind the object. At the same time a reference detector is used to record the radiation intensity from the x-ray tube.

3. The transmitted beam and the "reference beam" are both converted into electric current signals, I_n and I_R, respectively.

4. These output current signals are then converted into digital form by analog-to-digital converters (ADC).

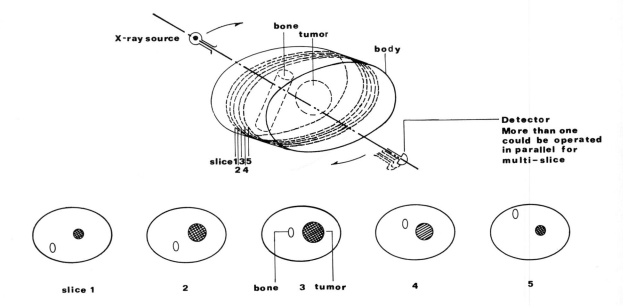

Figure 2–5. Computed tomography techniques on a body containing bone and tumor. (From Hounsfield, G.N.: Computerized transverse axial scanning (tomography). Part 1. Description of system. Br. Radiol., *46*:1016–1022, 1973. Reproduced by permission.)

    5. The digital data are then normalized and the logarithms calculated to generate *relative transmission values* (Hounsfield, 1973) where

$$\text{Relative transmission} = \log \frac{\text{intensity of x-rays at source}}{\text{intensity of x-rays at detector}}$$

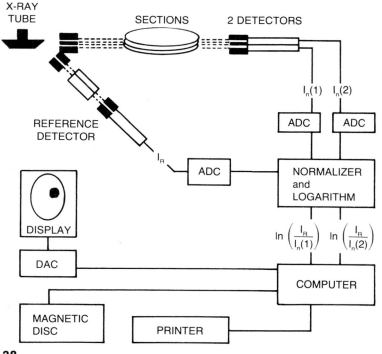

Figure 2–6. Essential components for the total acquisition of a CT image. See text for explanation. (From Phelps, M.E., Hoffman, E.J., Gado, M., and Ter-Pogossian, M.M.: Computerized transaxial transmission reconstruction tomography. *In* DeBlanc, H.R., Jr., and Sorenson, J.A. (Eds.): Non-Invasive Brain Imaging. New York, The Society of Nuclear Medicine, Inc., 1975. Reproduced by permission.)

6. The relative transmission values are sent to the computer, which uses a suitable program to reconstruct cross sections of the object.

7. The output from the computer (digital in form) can be sent to a line printer to produce a numerical print-out (Fig. 2–7), or . . .

8. The output can be put onto suitable storage devices (e.g., magnetic disk) for analysis of the information at a later time, or . . .

9. The output undergoes digital-to-analog conversion (DAC), after which it can be displayed on suitable devices (CRT display device) in varying shades of gray. (A color image is also possible.) The image can then be recorded by photographic means (Fig. 2–8).

In CT, the patient is first scanned using special motions of the x-ray tube and detectors. In the second step, which involves sampling, transmission values are obtained through the process given in step 5 above. In quantization, integers are assigned to the transmission values obtained as a result of sampling. These integers (gray levels) can be obtained as a numerical print-out (Fig. 2–7) or can be displayed as a gray scale (Fig. 2–8).

Distribution of Attenuation Values

To understand attentuation in CT, consider the following. When a homogeneous beam of x-rays passes through a uniform thickness of absorber, its attentuation (reduction in photon energy) follows an exponential law and is related to a coefficient (μ), referred to as the *linear attenuation coefficient*. The coefficient appears in the equation

$$I = I_0 e^{-\mu x}$$

where

$$I = \text{Transmitted photons}$$

$$I_0 = \text{Original number of incident photons}$$

$$x = \text{Absorber thickness}$$

$$e = \text{Euler's constant (2.718)}$$

$$\mu = \text{Linear attenuation coefficient}$$

The equation can be rewritten in the following manner:

$$\frac{I}{I_0} = e^{-\mu x}$$

$$= \ln \frac{I}{I_0} = -\mu x$$

$$= \ln \frac{I_0}{I} = \mu x$$

$$\mu = \frac{1}{x} \cdot \ln \frac{I_0}{I}$$

where ln is the natural logarithm, and μ is the only unknown quantity in the equation. Thus, by knowing I_0, I, and x, the value of μ can be obtained.

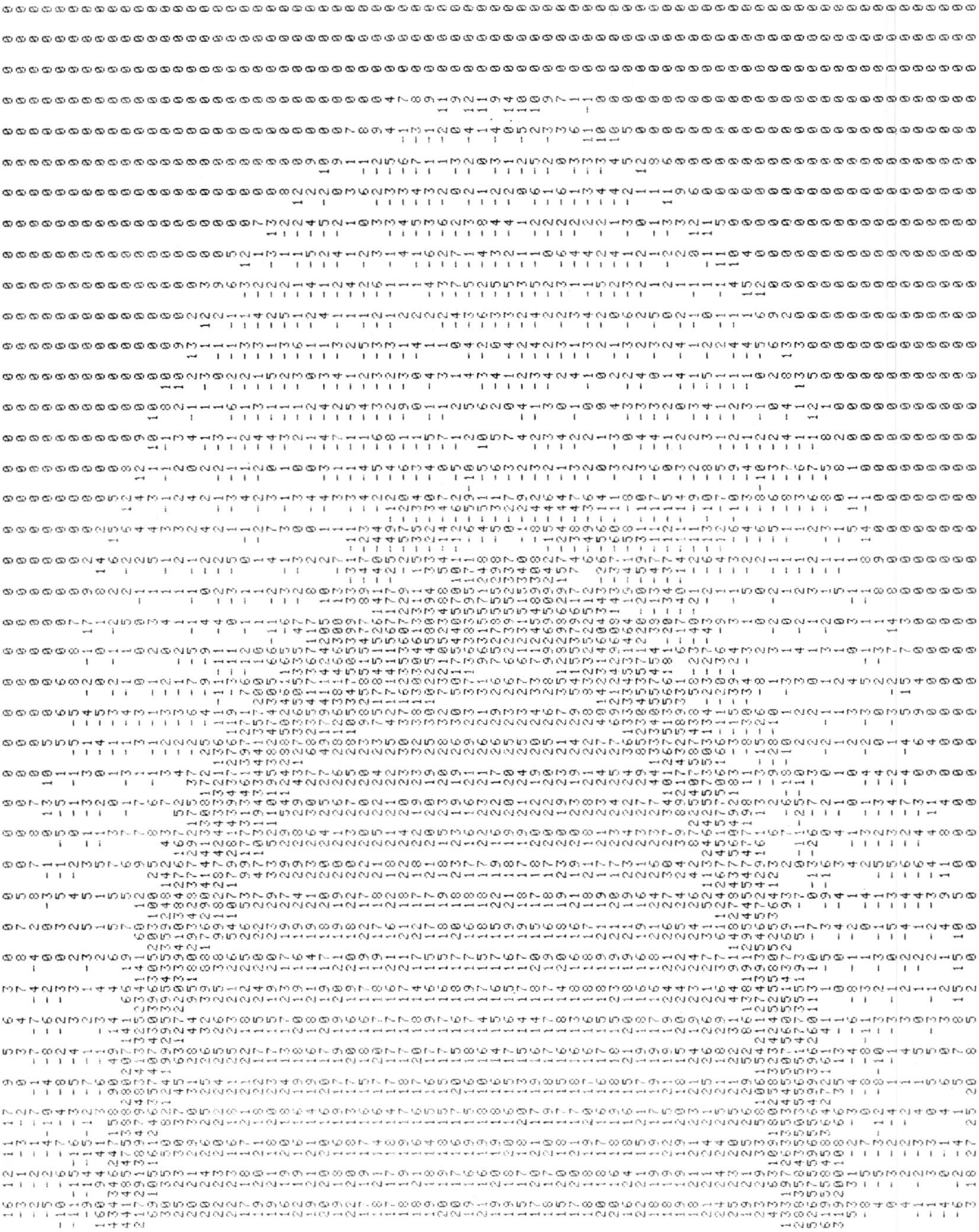

Figure 2-7. The appearance of the CT image on the line printer.

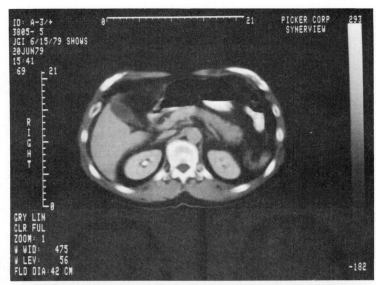

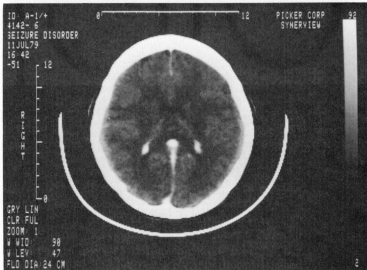

Figure 2–8. The appearance of the CT image on the television monitor. (Images provided by Picker International.)

Attenuation in CT depends on the effective atomic density (atoms/vol.), the atomic number (Z) of the absorber, and the photon energy. The x-rays interact by photoelectric and Compton effects. Photoelectric absorption occurs mainly in substances with high Z (bone, contrast media) and to a minimal extent in some soft tissues and substances with lower Z (McCullough, 1975; Phelps et al., 1975a). The Compton effect, on the other hand, occurs in soft tissues, and differences in density result in differences in the Compton interactions; thus, it is attributed primarily to density differences.

The distribution of attenuation values of clinical importance is shown in Figure 2–9. The values are established on a relative scale with the attenuation of water used as a reference. For example, on the first clinically useful CT scanner (EMI CT brain scanner), the values are established such that water is 0, while bone and air have values of +500 and −500, respectively. In order to

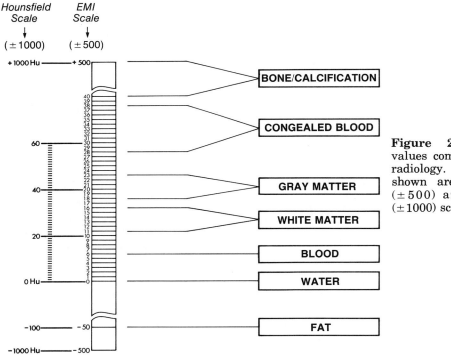

Figure 2–9. Absorption values common to clinical radiology. The values shown are for the EMI (±500) and Hounsfield (±1000) scales.

obtain more precision, a scale in which water is 0 and bone and air have values of +1000 and −1000 (Hounsfield scale) has been introduced.

In CT, the computer uses a series of digital numbers to reconstruct the image. These digital numbers are referred to as *CT numbers* (or currently, Hounsfield numbers), which are related to μ for various tissues in the patient. McCullough and Payne et al. (1976) have shown that

$$\text{CT Number} = \left[\frac{\mu - \mu_w}{\mu_w}\right] \cdot a$$

where μ = Attenuation coefficient of the measured tissue

μ_w = Attenuation coefficient of water

and a = Manufacturer's contrast factor.

Some typical values of a are 500 and 1000. In the original EMI CT scanner, the *contrast factor* (scaling factor) was 500; this gives a contrast scale of 0.2 per cent per CT number (Gado et al., 1977).

It is interesting to note that CT numbers were first referred to as *EMI numbers*. Recently, the scaling factor was increased twofold (i.e., 500 × 2), and hence new CT numbers are now referred to as *Hounsfield (H) units,* after the inventor. Today, H units are used on some scanners because of the advantage of expressing μ much more precisely (Alfidi and MacIntyre, 1976). The contrast scale with this system is 0.1 per cent per CT number (Gado et al., 1977).

One important point which deserves attention is that the Hounsfield unit is dependent on the photon energy, "since the attenuation coefficients of tissue and water may have different energy dependence" (Brooks and DiChiro, 1976).

Once CT numbers are obtained, it is essential to the diagnostician that this numerical image be converted to a gray scale image, which is more useful to him. Therefore, brightness levels (gray scale) corresponding to CT numbers must be established. This relationship (CT numbers to brightness level) is shown in Figure 2–10, where the upper (+1000) and the lower (−1000) limits of the scale represent white and black, respectively. All the other values represent varying shades of gray. The relationship between the CT numbers and shades of gray is variable and is referred to as "setting a window."

Number of Measurements

The number of measurements (sampling points) will primarily determine the spatial resolution of the final image. In order to obtain a spatial resolution of 1 mm., approximately 500 measurements are required across the object being scanned. More measurements would improve resolution but would require more time, more computation, and higher patient radiation dose.

kVp Technique

A high-voltage technique (for example, 120 kVp) is characteristic of CT imaging. The purpose of this, as pointed out by Phelps et al. (1975b) is

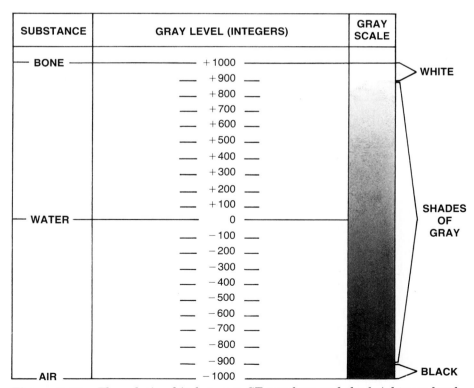

Figure 2–10. The relationship between CT numbers and the brightness level (gray scale) for the ±1000 scale.

threefold: "to produce a high transmitted beam flux at the detector, to reduce the contrast of skull relative to brain and to minimize energy-dependent variation in attenuation coefficients." These three reasons are important to ensure optimum detector response, to reduce artifacts due to changes in skull thickness which can conceal small changes in attenuation in soft tissues, and to minimize artifacts due to beam hardening effects (see Chap. 5), respectively (Phelps et al., 1975b).

SOME RELATED TERMINOLOGY

Voxels, Pixels, and Matrix

Since the x-ray beam has a finite width, attenuation coefficients will be reconstructed for very small volume elements in the object scanned. These volume elements are referred to as *voxels*. A typical volume element in CT currently measures 10 mm. in depth, 1.0 mm. in width, and 1.0 mm. in length. As the voxel size decreases, patient exposure increases to maintain good image

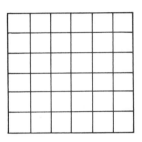

6 × 6 MATRIX
(36 PIXELS)

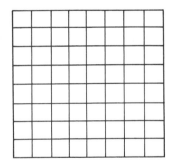

8 × 8 MATRIX
(64 PIXELS)

Figure 2–11. Three different matrix sizes. The number of image points (pixels) will increase with larger matrices.

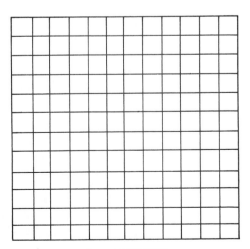

12 × 12 MATRIX
(144 PIXELS)

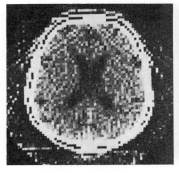 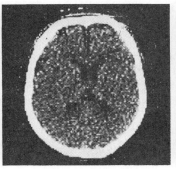 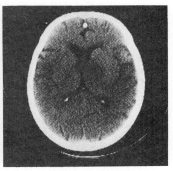

80 × 80 matrix   *128 × 128 matrix*   *256 × 256 matrix*

Figure 2–12.   The effect of three different matrix sizes on the resolution of the CT image. (From Scharl, P., Weckesser, W.D., and Peter, F.: Problems in the display of CT images by the use of television and photography. Electromedica, 2:62–65, 1979. Reproduced by permission.)

quality. The voxel (always in the object) is displayed as little squares or picture elements on the CT image display. The picture elements are called *pixels*.

A *matrix* (computer matrix) is an array of pixels arranged in two dimensions (rows and columns). Figure 2–11 shows four different sizes of matrices. In CT, as the number of points (pixels) increases (i.e., the larger the matrix), the quality of the image improves. This effect is clearly demonstrated in Figure 2–12. A matrix of attenuation coefficients for each section of the object scanned is produced by the computer and can be printed out directly using a high-speed print-out device.

In Figure 2–13, a representation of a voxel on a computer matrix is shown.

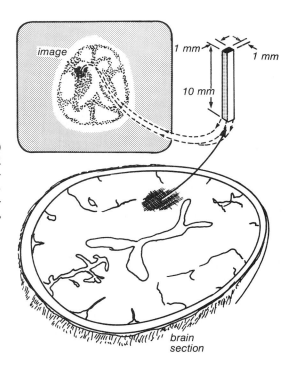

Figure 2–13.   A representation of a voxel (1.0 mm. × 1.0 mm. × 10 mm.) that is displayed as a pixel on a computer matrix. (From Ter-Pogossian, M. M.: Physics and equipment. *In* Felson, B. (Ed.): Computerized Cranial Tomography. New York, Grune and Stratton, Inc., 1977. Reproduced by permission.)

TECHNOLOGY — ESSENTIAL CHARACTERISTICS

Since the introduction of the first EMI CT unit, many new scanners for both brain and whole body have become commercially available. There have also been rapid changes in the technology and the performance characteristics of the scanners, as these ultimately affect the method of data collection for CT images. Because of this, a simple categorization of CT equipment has evolved (Brownell, 1976). This categorization is based on the scanning mode and the number of detectors (method of data collection) used in each category.

To date (1981), four categories of clinically useful CT scanners have been identified:

a. First-generation: *Single x-ray beam — translate/rotate.*
b. Second-generation: *Multiple x-ray beams — translate/rotate.*
c. Third-generation: *Fan beam — rotary motion of tube and detector.*
d. Fourth-generation: *Stationary detector array with rotary fan beam.*

First-generation CT Scanners

In first-generation CT equipment, the method of data collection is based on a *rotate/translate principle,* in which a single-beam x-ray tube and one or two detectors translate and rotate in 1° increments for 180° around the patient's head. The scanning method is usually referred to as *rectilinear pencil beam scanning.* Figure 2–14 illustrates the method of data collection for first-generation CT scanners. As the x-ray tube translates across the object, a series of readings of transmitted intensity is obtained. The process is repeated when the x-ray tube and detector(s) are rotated through angular increments of 1°.

To produce one complete scan of the object requires approximately 4.5 to 5.5 minutes. Therefore, if more cross sections are required, the examination time will be increased.

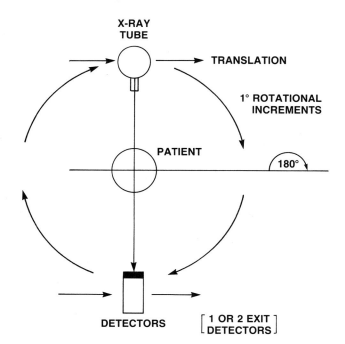

Figure 2–14. Rectilinear pencil beam scanning typical of first-generation CT scanners, based on the rotate/translate principle.

Since the x-ray tube is mechanically coupled to the detector system, the scanning process involves the following:

a. The tube and detector move across the object in a straight line and then stop.

b. The tube and detector rotate 1°, start again, and move across the object — this time in the opposite direction — and then stop.

c. This process — translate, stop, rotate, translate, stop, rotate — is repeated 180 times.

This method is obviously time-consuming. Originally, one detector was used, but with the introduction of a second detector two scan slices can now be obtained simultaneously within the 4.5 to 5.5 minutes. The obvious limitations of first-generation CT equipment are that (a) scan time is too long for the patient to hold his breath or to remain perfectly immobile during the scanning process, and (b) patient throughput is restricted.

Other limitations are also present, but these will become apparent in later discussions.

Second-generation CT Scanners

Second-generation scanners employ a large number of detectors and a modified x-ray beam (several pencil beams) from a single x-ray tube. Like first-generation scanners, they are based on the rotate/translate principle but use a *rectilinear multiple pencil beam scanning technique*. Since the number of detectors has increased, the angular increment is larger.

The principle of second-generation CT scanners is illustrated in Figure 2–15. The x-ray tube and detectors rotate with successive translation to produce an increase in the data set to be collected. The scan time for second-generation scanners is shorter and ranges from about 20 seconds to 3.5 minutes for some equipment. Generally, the time decrease is inversely

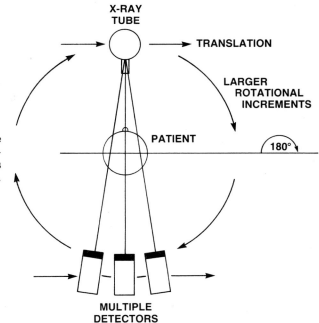

Figure 2–15. Rectilinear multiple pencil beam scanning used in second-generation CT scanners. The method is based on the rotate/translate principle.

proportional to the number of detectors (Brownell, 1976). The more detectors, the shorter the total scan time.

The advantages of second-generation equipment are obvious. Since the total scan time is decreased, artifacts such as image blurring due to respiratory motion are eliminated. However, "the density and spatial resolution are not appreciably different" (Brownell, 1976).

Third-generation CT Scanners

Third-generation scanners offer an even shorter scan time than do second-generation scanners. The fundamental principle of third-generation units is shown in Figure 2–16. The principle is based on a *continuously rotating pulsed fan beam scanning technique*. The CT image is obtained by using a pure fan beam of radiation and multiple detectors. This principle enables data collection within five to ten seconds. This scan time precludes artifacts due to respiratory motion.

Fourth-generation CT Scanners

This generation of scanners consists of multiple fixed detectors that form a ring around the object. The x-ray source moves around the object through 360°. Such a system is illustrated in Figure 2–17. The beam geometry describes a wide fan. On scanning, the fan beam strikes the detectors as it rotates and the detector signals are recorded during the rotation. Scan times of 2 to 10 seconds can be achieved with this design.

Fifth-generation CT Scanners

A further reduction in scan speed would require multiple x-ray sources and more detectors. Already such a scanner is being developed under the direction of Dr. E. Woods of the Mayo Clinic. The system consists essentially of

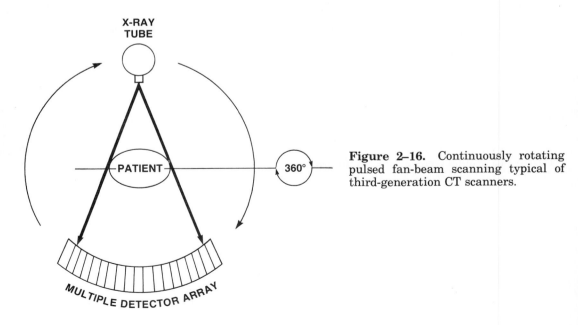

Figure 2–16. Continuously rotating pulsed fan-beam scanning typical of third-generation CT scanners.

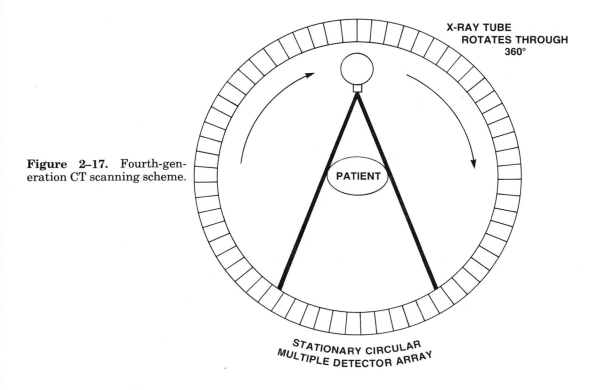

Figure 2–17. Fourth-generation CT scanning scheme.

multiple x-ray tubes and multiple detectors. Such a unit will be used to image a three-dimensional section of the heart and reduce artifacts due to cardiac rhythm (Alfidi and Haaga, 1976). A further description of this scanner will be given in Chapter 9.

Table 2–1 summarizes the four categories of CT scanners with respect to some prototypes, number of detectors, type of radiation beam, and scan time.

TABLE 2–1. CATEGORIES OF CT EQUIPMENT WITH RESPECT TO SOME COMMERCIALLY AVAILABLE UNITS

GENERATION	PROTOTYPE	NUMBER OF DETECTORS PER SLICE	TYPE OF RADIATION BEAM	SCAN TIME
First-generation	a. EMI brain scanner b. ACTA	1	Single	~5 min.
Second-generation	EMI CT 5005	30	Multiple	~20 sec.
Third-generation	a. General Electric CT/T body scanner b. Siemens Somatom 2	260 or 520 511	Pulsed-fan Pulsed-fan	4.8 sec. and 9.6 sec. 5 sec. and 10 sec.
Fourth-generation	a. Picker Synerview b. Pfizer 450 c. EMI 7070	600 600 1150	Continuous fan Continuous fan Continuous fan	2–10 sec. 5–10 sec. 2–10 sec.

CT / 2

SUMMARY/REFERENCES/BIBLIOGRAPHY/REVIEW QUESTIONS

Summary

1. CT is a new x-ray imaging technique used in clinical radiology, the principles of which may be traced back to several mathematical and related developments.

2. It was independently developed by Godfrey Hounsfield of EMI in England. For this development, he recently shared the Nobel Prize in Medicine and Physiology with physics professor Alan Cormack of Tufts University in the United States. Professor Cormack initially worked out mathematical solutions to problems in CT.

3. The most conspicuous difference between CT and conventional x-ray imaging is that CT images cross-sectional anatomy. CT also overcomes several limitations (such as superimposition of structures) imposed by conventional radiography and tomography.

4. In CT, the object is scanned by a highly collimated x-ray beam. Special detectors, which are used to measure transmission of x-rays through the object, convert the radiation beam into electric signals, which are in turn converted to digital information.

5. These measurements are used to calculate absorption values (attenuation values) of various structures within the object.

6. The values are then utilized by the computer to calculate CT numbers. These CT numbers are used in reconstructing a picture of cross-sectional anatomy that can be displayed as a numerical print-out or as a gray-scale image.

7. For successful imaging, many x-ray transmission readings must be obtained from the object. This is accomplished by using special movements of the x-ray tube and detectors.

8. The volume of tissue imaged in CT is referred to as a voxel, which is displayed on a television monitor as a pixel or picture element. Rows and columns of pixels form a matrix. Generally, the larger the matrix, the larger the number of pixels.

9. CT equipment currently falls into four categories. This categorization is based on the scanning mode and the number of detectors used by each.

10. First-generation CT equipment is based on a rotate/translate principle using a single pencil beam of radiation and one or two detectors.

11. Second-generation scanners use the same rotate/translate principle, multiple x-ray beams, and multiple detectors (up to 30).

12. Third-generation CT scanners use a continuously rotating pulsed fan-beam of radiation, with a detector array (greater than second-generation scanners) system.

13. Fourth-generation CT scanners make use of a fixed circular array of detectors and an x-ray source which moves around the object.

14. The development of fifth-generation CT scanners that make use of multiple x-ray sources is now in progress, and they will be available in the near future.

References

Alfidi, R. J., and Haaga, J. R.: Computed tomography of the body. A new horizon. Postgrad. Med., 59:133–136, 1976.

Alfidi, R. J., and MacIntyre, W. J.: Computed tomography standardization. Radiology, 119:743–744, 1976.

Bocage, E. M.: Pat. No. 536,464, Paris, France. *Quoted in* Massiot, J.: History of tomography. Medicamundi, 19:106–115, 1974.

Brooks, R. A., and DiChiro, G.: Principles of computer assisted tomography (CAT) in radiographic and radioisotopic imaging. Phys. Med. Biol., 21:689–732, 1976.

Brownell, G. L.: Personal communication, 1976.

Gado, M., Eichling, J., and Currie, M.: Quantitative aspects of CT images. *In* Norman, D., Korobkin, M., and Newton, T. (Eds.): Computer Tomography. St. Louis, The C.V. Mosby Company, 1977.

Hounsfield, G. N.: Computerized transverse axial scanning (tomography). Part 1. Description of the system. Br. J. Radiol., 46:1016–1022, 1973.

Marshall, C. H.: Principles of computed tomography. Postgrad. Med., 59:105–109, 1976.

McCullough, E. C.: Photon attenuation in CT. Med. Phys., 2:307–320, 1975.

McCullough, E. C.: Personal communication, 1976.

McCullough, E. C., Payne, J. T., et al.: Performance evaluation and quality assurance of computed tomography scanners with illustrations from EMI, ACTA and DELTA scanners. Radiology, 120:173–188, 1976.

Phelps, M. E., Gado, M. H., and Hoffman, E. J.: Correlation of effective atomic number and electron density with attenuation coefficients measured with polychromatic x-ray. Radiology, 117:585–588, 1975a.

Phelps, M. E., Hoffman, E. J., Gado, M., and Ter-Pogossian, M. M.: Computerized transaxial transmission reconstruction tomography. *In* DeBlanc, H. R., Jr., and Sorenson, J. A. (Eds.): Non-Invasive Brain Imaging. New York, The Society of Nuclear Medicine, Inc., 1975b.

Scharl, P., Weckesser, W. D., and Peter, F.: Problems in the display of CT images by the use of television and photography. Electromedica, 2:62–65, 1979.

Ter-Pogossian, M. M., et al.: The extraction of the yet unused wealth of information in diagnostic radiology. Radiology, 113:515–520, 1974.

Ter-Pogossian, M. M.: Physics and equipment. *In* Felson, B. (Ed.): Computerized Cranial Tomography. New York, Grune and Stratton, Inc., 1977.

Vallebona, A.: Radiography with great enlargement (micro radiography) and a technical method for radiographic dissociation of the shadow. Radiology, 17:340–341, 1931.

Bibliography

Hounsfield, G. N.: Computerized transverse axial scanning (tomography). Part 1. Description of the system. Br. J. Radiol., 46:1016–1022, 1973.

Hounsfield, G. N.: Historical notes on computerized axial tomography. J. Can. Assoc. Radiol., 27:1976.

Seeram, E.: Computed tomography. An overview. Radiol. Technol., 49:491–496, 1978.

Seeram, E.: Computed tomography: Physical basis and technology. X-ray Focus, 17:34–39, 1979.

Review Questions

1. CT is a new technique in x-ray imaging that does not:
   (a) Use a computer to reconstruct cross-sectional images of an object.
   (b) Use mathematical methods to reconstruct cross-sectional images of an object.
   (c) Use special detectors to detect x-rays that have passed through an object at multiple angles.
   (d) Use x-ray film as the image receptor.

2. CT is not synonymous with:
   (a) Computer assisted tomography.
   (b) Reconstructive tomography.
   (c) Transaxial emission tomography.
   (d) Computerized axial tomography.

3. Which of the following independently developed a method of separating out tissue densities using an external beam of radiation?
    (a) Kuhl
    (b) Oldendorf
    (c) Ambrose
    (d) Hounsfield

4. Who developed the first whole body CT scanner?
    (a) Hounsfield
    (b) Ambrose
    (c) Ledley
    (d) General Electric Company

5. The limitations imposed by focal plane tomography are removed by CT through:
    (a) The use of a highly collimated beam of x-rays and special detectors and passing the x-ray beam only through the cross section of interest.
    (b) The use of special sodium iodide detectors only.
    (c) The use of a computer.
    (d) The use of special motions of x-ray tube and detectors.

6. A voxel is:
    (a) A picture element of the television monitor.
    (b) A volume of tissue in the object.
    (c) An array of numbers arranged in rows and columns.
    (d) Another term for attenuation coefficients.

7. In CT, the relative transmission value to be used for reconstruction of any material within each slice of the object is given to be:
    (a) The log of the ratio of the intensity of x-rays at the source to the intensity of x-rays at the detector.
    (b) The log of the ratio of the intensity of x-rays at the detector to the intensity at the source.
    (c) The ratio of the intensity of x-rays at the source to the intensity of x-rays at the detector.
    (d) The ratio of intensity of x-rays at the detector to the intensity of x-rays at the source.

8. The decrease in scan time in CT is attributed to the:
    (a) Number of detectors.
    (b) Type of detectors.
    (c) Type of x-ray tube.
    (d) Type of rectification.

9. In CT, the decrease in scan time is:
    (a) Inversely proportional to the number of detectors.
    (b) Directly proportional to the number of detectors.
    (c) Not related to the detectors.
    (d) Inversely proportional to the number of radiation beams.

10. The number of slices that can be obtained from an object of diameter D is:
    (a) Directly proportional to the diameter and inversely proportional to the width of the slice.
    (b) Directly proportional to the diameter times the width of the slice.
    (c) Inversely proportional to the diameter only.
    (d) Directly proportional to the width of the slice and inversely proportional to the diameter.

11. The number of pixels in an 80×80 matrix is:
    (a) 160
    (b) 640
    (c) 6400
    (d) 80

12. If the linear attenuation coefficient for bone and water are 0.380 and 0.190, respectively, and the scaling factor of the scanner is 1000, the CT number for air is:
    (a) $+1000$
    (b) -1000
    (c) $+380$
    (d) $+190$

13. If the attenuation coefficients for bone and water are 0.380 and 0.190, respectively, and the scaling factor of the CT scanner is 500, the CT number for bone is:
    (a) 0
    (b) -500
    (c) $+500$
    (d) $+1000$

14. Which generation of CT scanners is based on the translate/rotate principle using a single x-ray beam?
    (a) First-generation
    (b) Second-generation
    (c) Third-generation
    (d) Fourth-generation

15. Which of the following is characteristic of fourth-generation CT scanners?
    (a) Five minutes to complete scan
    (b) Stationary detectors with rotating fan-beam of x-rays
    (c) Rotation of x-ray tube and detectors with fan-beam of radiation
    (d) Multiple x-ray sources

16. Which of the following is true of second-generation CT scanners?
    (a) 30 detectors/slice, multiple radiation beams, and about 20 sec. scan time
    (b) 260 detectors/slice, pulsed fan-beam of radiation, and 4.8 sec. scan time
    (c) 520 detectors/slice, pulsed fan-beam of radiation, and 9.6 sec. scan time
    (d) 600 detectors/slice, continuous fan-beam of radiation, and 2 to 10 sec. scan time

17. Which of the following influences the value of the Hounsfield unit?
    (a) The energy of the radiation beam
    (b) The scanning motion
    (c) The number of detectors
    (d) The number of slices

CT

CHAPTER 3

X-RAY SOURCES, FILTRATION, COLLIMATION, AND DETECTORS

In his initial experiments he used low energy gamma rays which he scanned across blocks of perspex rotated on a modified lathe bench, onto crystal detectors.*

EMI CENTRAL RESEARCH LABS (1977)

X-RAY SOURCES

SOURCE REQUIREMENTS

The radiation source requirement in CT depends on two factors: (a) radiation attenuation, which is a function of the energy of the radiation beam, the atomic number and density of the absorber, and the total object thickness, and (b) the quantity of the radiation desired for transmission.

Although initial experiments in CT were done using monochromatic radiation sources, the use of these sources in clinical CT is not practical

---

*G. N. Hounsfield.

because of the low-radiation intensity rate. Additional limitations include large source size, low source strength, and high cost.

At present, CT technology utilizes conventional x-ray tubes because they provide the high-radiation intensities necessary for clinical high-contrast CT scanning (McCullough and Payne, 1977).

TYPES OF X-RAY TUBES

Two types of x-ray tubes are used today in CT scanners:

1. *Fixed-anode* oil-cooled x-ray tubes of the industrial type. They can be energized continuously and are based on the line focus principle. Their basic design incorporates a tungsten target with a typical 20° angle of bevel and a focal spot size of 2×16 mm. The anode and cathode structures are encased in an evacuated Pyrex glass envelope. The total filtration of these tubes may range from 3.5 mm. Al to 7.5 mm. Al for some scanners (McCullough and Payne, 1977).

The disadvantages of these tubes are (a) that continuous operation will result in high noise due to statistical variations in the number of detected photons (for some studies) and not enough photons per view, and (b) that large focal spot tubes (without proper collimation) will increase patient exposure owing to greater penumbral overlap as compared to small focal spots.

2. *Rotating-anode* x-ray tubes. Several manufacturers incorporate rotating-anode tubes in their "sub-10-sec" CT machines. These tubes are air-cooled and may be pulsed in operation or run continuously for short times. The heat storage capacities of the anode and tube housing limit their use on a continuous basis. The operate at tube currents to about 600 mA. Patient exposure is limited because their small focal spots (for example, 0.6 mm.) decrease penumbral overlap for multiple scans.

Pulsing the x-ray beam during operation (as the tube moves continuously around the patient) allows for time to recalibrate the electronics between pulses. Depending on the patient's size, the pulse length can be changed to (a) increase the detector response and (b) increase the number of photons in order to reduce noise (McCullough and Payne, 1977).

It should be noted that to prolong tube life of rotating-anode tubes used on a continuous basis, it would be worthwhile to allow sufficient time for the tube to cool.

FILTRATION

The purpose of a filter in CT is essentially twofold:

1. To absorb low-energy x-rays (soft radiation) that do not contribute to the acquisition of the CT image. By doing this, patient dose is reduced and the beam quality increases (the beam becomes "harder").

2. To shape the energy distribution across the radiation beam to produce uniform beam hardening when x-rays pass through the filter and the object.

To understand No. 2, consider the circular object shown in Figure 3–1. The attenuation will be different in sections A, B, and C, and so will be the penetration in sections B and C, with increased penetration in section C. This is a result of absorption of the soft radiation in sections A and B. The total

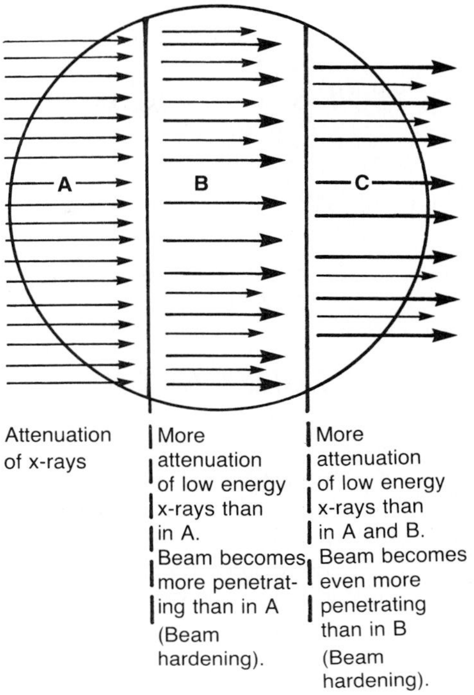

Figure 3–1. The attenuation of radiation through a circular object. The beam becomes more penetrating (harder) in Section C because of differences in attenuation in Sections A and B. The heavier arrows indicate less attenuation and more penetrating rays.

Attenuation of x-rays

More attenuation of low energy x-rays than in A. Beam becomes more penetrating than in A (Beam hardening).

More attenuation of low energy x-rays than in A and B. Beam becomes even more penetrating than in B (Beam hardening).

result is referred to as *hardening of the beam.* Since the detector system does not respond to beam hardening effects (for a circular object), the problem can be solved by introducing additional filtration into the beam. The shape of the filter is such that it conforms to the shape of the object being scanned (General Electric, 1978).

In the original EMI scanner, this problem was solved by using a square water box where the object (the patient's head) within the box represented a part of the square box. Figure 3–2 shows two filters that are placed between the x-ray tube and object to reduce the dynamic range of the electronics (analog-to-digital converters), by shaping the beam to produce uniform beam hardening. Added filters for body and head CT scanning differ significantly in their size and shape.

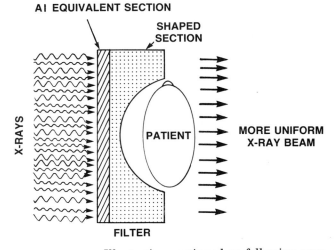

Figure 3–2. Added filters for beam shaping in CT (see text for explanation).

Illustration continued on following page

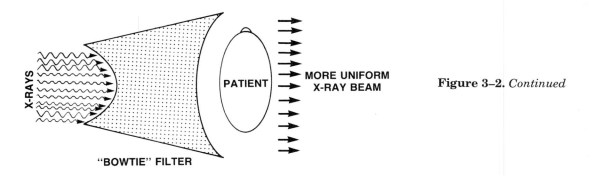

Figure 3–2. *Continued*

COLLIMATION

In any x-ray imaging system, collimation is important, since it influences patient dose and image quality by limiting the beam only to the field of interest and reducing the amount of scattered radiation.

In CT, collimation can be a complex subject and therefore only the necessary details will be pointed out here. The basic collimation scheme in a CT system is shown in Figure 3–3. Two kinds are apparent, the x-ray tube collimator and the detector collimator. From Figure 3–3, it can be seen that their alignment must be accurate.

THE X-RAY TUBE COLLIMATOR

The design of the x-ray tube collimator system is important, since there is a penumbra effect associated with the size of the focal spot. In general, the

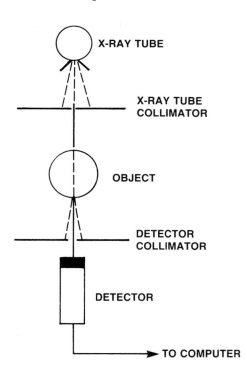

Figure 3–3. A typical collimation scheme in a CT system.

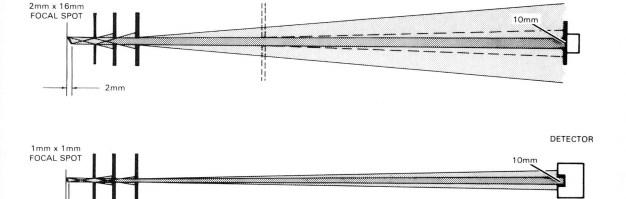

Figure 3–4. The effect of focal spot size on collimator design. The dotted collimator blade would have to be positioned at the point indicated if the same beam geometry as the smaller focal spot size is to the obtained. (Courtesy of General Electric, Medical Systems Division, 1978.)

larger the focal spot size, the more complicated the collimator design, in order to reduce radiation dose and produce a beam of the same geometry as that of a smaller focal spot. This can be seen in Figure 3–4.

It is also important to note the intensity profile of the collimated beam (Fig. 3–5) because the design requirements for CT collimators, as set up by the Bureau of Radiological Health (USA), are stated in terms of beam intensity profiles.

DETECTOR COLLIMATORS

These collimators are located in front of the detectors and play a role in eliminating scattered rays. Two detector collimation schemes are shown in Figure 3–6. The apparent difference is in the spacing of the apertures. Because of this, the design scheme in *B* uses the radiation beam more efficiently, since it has about three times as many detectors as *A*.

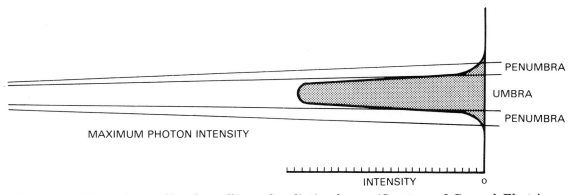

Figure 3–5. Intensity profile of a collimated radiation beam. (Courtesy of General Electric, Medical Systems Division, 1978.)

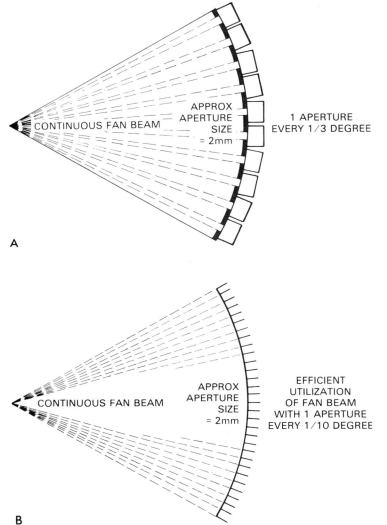

A

Figure 3–6. Detector collimation schemes for second *(A)* and third *(B)* generation CT systems. See text for explanation. (Courtesy of General Electric, Medical Systems Division, 1978.)

B

In conclusion, the following points should be noted:

1. The collimator aperture width determines the thickness of the CT section (slice thickness). This is specified by numerical values, the most typical being 3 mm., 5 mm., 8 mm., 10 mm., and 13 mm. These values refer to the slice thicknesses in the reconstructed image.

2. The criteria for selection of collimation are based on the trade-off of pixel width, scan noise, patient dose, and slice thickness.

3. Collimation does not determine pixel width. Such size is related to the computer program (Christensen et al., 1978).

4. The slice thickness is generally greater than the width of the pixel (McCullough and Payne, 1977).

RESEARCH FINDINGS

Thomas et al. (1978) investigated the different types of collimators in terms of performance and clinical application. More specifically, the purpose of the study was to investigate the advantages and disadvantages associated with collimation in the EMI MK1 brain scanner and especially to look at the "effects involved with areas within the brain and not within the orbital regions" (Thomas et al., 1978).

The following points were made by Thomas et al. (1978) in summarizing their study:

> a. The small collimators do provide a gain in spatial resolution in the Z direction (perpendicular to the image plane), which allows a more precise determination of small lesion thickness and, subsequently, of lesion volume. No direct gain in spatial resolution is achieved in the X-Y plane (image plane) through the use of the small collimators; however, through the associated reduction of volume averaging, edge of definition in the X-Y plane is improved and a better definition of lesion boundaries may be obtained.

> b. Simple volume-averaging theory and standard-deviation considerations indicate that little gain in diagnostic information will be obtained with the small collimators if the lesion density is close to that of the surrounding brain tissue. For brain tissue with an EMI No. of 15, the lesion should have a true EMI No. greater than 30 if the 3-mm. collimators are to be of substantial value. Consequently, the small collimators will be of greater value under contrast conditions.

This is due to lower photon statistics with a thin slice and thus higher image noise.

> c. Clinical and phantom studies have indicated that the 3-mm. collimators may improve visualization of lesions that are close to the skull curvature through reduction of the so-called "increased density peripheral zone" artifact.

It has generally been observed that thinner cuts result in less beam hardening artifacts.

DETECTORS

The purpose of the detection system in CT is to gather information by measuring the x-ray transmission through the object. The detector is an integral component in the total system and therefore should possess certain properties in order to maximize performance.

PROPERTIES OF DETECTORS

Several properties of detectors are identified in Table 3–1, the most important ones being *efficiency, response time,* and *stability* (McCullough and Payne, 1977).

Efficiency refers to *quantum detection efficiency.* This is the efficiency with which the detector detects x-ray photons. It is an expression of the percentage of photons incident on the detector that results in a detector signal. On the other hand, the energy conversion in the detector is based on two principles. Essentially, some detectors convert the x-ray energy into light energy, which is in turn converted into electrical pulses, while other detectors convert the x-ray energy directly into electrical pulses. These conversion events will be discussed in the next section.

**TABLE 3–1. SEVERAL IMPORTANT PROPERTIES OF DETECTORS
USED IN CT TECHNOLOGY***

Cost/detector
Dynamic range
   Noise
   Saturation
Efficiency (preferably high)
Linearity (or reproducible response)
Response time (large flux changes)
Size
Stability (between calibrations)
Weak energy sensitivity (for less than 100% efficiency)

*From McCullough, E. C., and Payne, J. T.: X-ray transmission computed tomography. Med. Phys., *4*(2): 85–98, 1977. Reproduced by permission.

Stability pertains to the steadiness of the detector response. If a detector system is not stable, frequent calibrations are necessary to correct for the instability and make it possible to produce artifact-free images. Response time refers to the speed with which the detectors can detect an x-ray event and recover in order to detect another x-ray event. The response time of detectors should be very short (microseconds) to avoid problems such as afterglow or detector pile-up.

TYPES OF DETECTORS

At present, detectors used in CT fall into two classes: (a) scintillation detectors, and (b) gas ionization detectors. A typical *scintillation detector* (e.g., one used in a translate/rotate CT scanner) is the sodium iodide (NaI) or cesium iodide (CsI) crystal coupled to a photomultiplier tube. This arrangement is shown in Figure 3–7. When x-rays are absorbed by the crystal, flashes of light (scintillations) are produced. The light is directed to a photomultiplier tube. Here the light strikes a photocathode, releasing electrons. These electrons in turn cascade through a series of dynodes carefully positioned within the tube and maintained at different potentials. Upon striking the first dynode, more

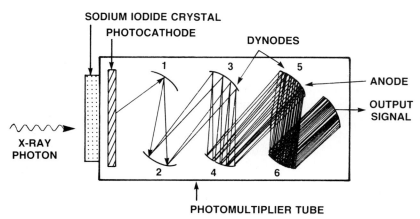

Figure 3–7. Schematic of a scintillation detector (see text for explanation).

electrons are knocked off and are then accelerated to fall upon the second dynode, which in turn emits more electrons than the first dynode. This action continues until the last dynode is reached. By this electron amplification process, a large number of electrons is produced, generally 10^6 or more. This number constitutes the output signal of the detector.

There are two points to note about scintillation detectors: (a) the amount of light produced in the crystals is directly proportional to the energy of the absorbed x-rays; and (b) the number of electrons emitted from the photocathode is proportional to the amount of light falling upon it.

Today a variety of crystals is available, including calcium fluoride (CaF_2) and bismuth germanate (BGO). These do not exhibit afterglow, a problem typical of NaI detectors. Another crystal that has been used is cesium iodide (CsI).

Another type of CT detector utilizes the *gas ionization* principle. To improve the detector efficiency, xenon gas is pressurized to about 20 atmospheres. This type of detector system is usually common to third-generation scanners.

Figure 3–8 shows a schematic of a xenon detector (for one type of scanner). It consists of tungsten plates (electrodes) carefully positioned so that they act as electron collection plates inside a sea of pressurized xenon. When a beam of radiation falls within an individual cell of the detector, ionization of the gas occurs. The positive ions migrate to the negatively charged plate, while the negative ions are attracted to the positively charged plate. The signal current varies directly with the number of x-ray photons absorbed.

Currently, both types of detectors are being used. In the future one may also see the appearance of solid-state detectors.

The advantages and disadvantages of the NaI and xenon CT detectors are presented in Table 3–2.

TABLE 3–2.   ADVANTAGES AND DISADVANTAGES OF CT DETECTORS

DETECTORS	ADVANTAGES	DISADVANTAGES
Sodium iodide crystal and photomultiplier tube	High detection efficiency; e.g., for a 1 in. crystal, the detection efficiency is ~100% at 70 keV (McCullough and Payne, 1978).	Afterglow Restricted dynamic range
Calcium fluoride (CaF_2)	No afterglow	Less detection efficiency than NaI; e.g., in a 1 in. crystal, the detection efficiency is about 62% (McCullough and Payne, 1978).
Bismuth germanate (BGO)	No afterglow High detection efficiency	Low light output
Xenon	Simple and more compact than NaI No afterglow	Inefficiency (low absorption efficiency — some photons pass through chamber without being detected) Stability problems Response time

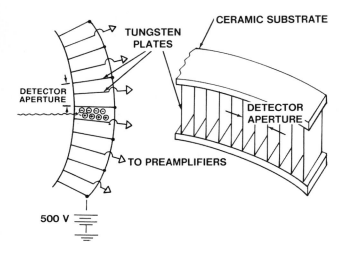

Figure 3–8. Schematic of xenon detector used in a CT system. See text for explanation. (Courtesy of General Electric, Medical Systems Division, 1978.)

RESEARCH FINDINGS

Brooks and DiChiro (1978) have investivated a *split-detector system* for use in CT. The study was undertaken to determine whether the technique was practical to acquire CT images as is possible with the *dual-energy method*. In the dual-energy method, scans are taken using two different energy levels, one at 100 kVp and the other at 140 kVp, since energy discrimination is a function of the effective atomic number and the chemical composition of the absorber.

The split-detector system used in the study is shown in Figure 3–9. Two scintillation detectors (NaI and CaF_2 coupled to photomultiplier tubes) are used to obtain information. The first detector (CaF_2) detects primarily low-energy x-rays, while the second one (NaI) detects the remainder of the beam.

The results of this study indicate the following:

a. With a split-detector system, it is possible to obtain two CT images at the same time (scanning only once).

b. Energy discrimination of the split-detector system is possibly better than the dual-energy method.

c. This system may be helpful in discriminating low-contrast substances "when the attenuation level is close to that of normal tissue" (Brooks and DiChiro, 1978).

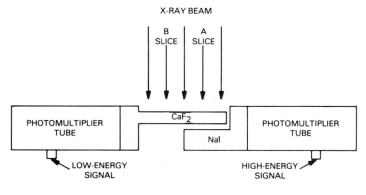

Figure 3–9. The split-detector system. (From Brooks, R.A., and DiChiro, G.: Split-detector computed tomography — a preliminary report. Radiology, *126*: 255–257, 1978. Reproduced by permission.)

Another interesting study is one by Beinglass et al. (1980), who investigated the feasibility of mercuric iodide (HgI_2) for use as a semiconductor x-ray detector in CT. Their results indicate that HgI_2 may be useful as a detector in CT, since it has a high detection efficiency, functions at room temperature, and has a stable response. These detectors, however, do present disadvantages such as the problem of having a long "memory" (afterglow).

THE USE OF INFORMATION FROM THE DETECTOR

When radiation falls upon the detector, a current signal is produced which undergoes electronic amplification. The acquisition of signals for the entire patient cross section (view) in a translate/rotate system is shown in Figure 3–10. The figure also illustrates how the amplitude of the signal is produced. The output signal from the detector amplifier is analog in form, and hence the next step involves converting it into a digital number, to be used by the computer for image reconstruction.

Essentially, analog-to-digital conversion involves assigning a number to the analog signal with a total range large enough to include the magnitude of any analog signal encountered in the study. This is illustrated in Figure 3–11.

The generation of the output signal in a rotate-only CT system is shown in Figure 3–12. The steps are the same for analog-to-digital conversion.

Finally, Table 3–3 presents a comparison of the criteria for data acquisition (detector and electronics) and response time of translate/rotate, non-pulsed, rotate-only, and pulsed rotate-only systems.

TABLE 3–3. A COMPARISON OF CRITERIA FOR DATA ACQUISITION (DETECTOR AND ELECTRONICS) AND RESPONSE TIME FOR THREE TYPES OF CT SYSTEMS*

CRITERIA	TRANSLATE/ROTATE	NON-PULSED, ROTATE ONLY	PULSED, ROTATE ONLY
Data collection per view	Each view is generated ray sum by ray sum or data point by data point as the mechanical system moves in a linear translation.	Each view is generated with the simultaneous detector element sampling over a referenced period of time determined by the speed of rotation.	Each view is generated with the simultaneous detector element output during the x-ray "on" pulse (usually 2 to 3 milliseconds).
Response speed per view	Approximately 1 sec. to 15 sec. depending on the speed of the scanner.	Approximately 10 milliseconds would be needed, depending upon the number of views and the speed of the rotation.	1 millisecond to 6 milliseconds, synchronous with the pulsing of the x-ray system.

*Courtesy of General Electric Company, Medical Systems Division, 1978.

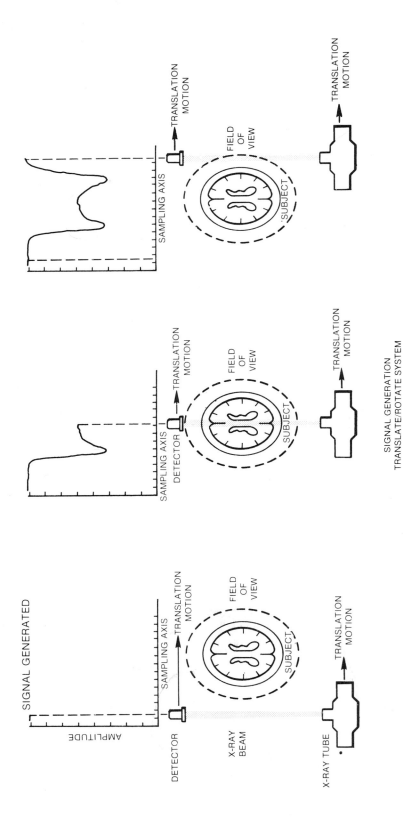

Figure 3-10. Generation of a current signal in a CT system. Signal generated for one translation. (Courtesy of General Electric, Medical Systems Division, 1978.)

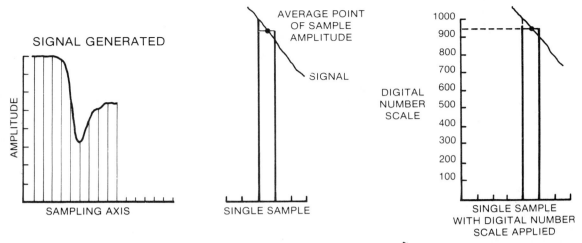

Figure 3–11. Analog-to-digital conversion of an output signal in CT. (Courtesy of General Electric, Medical Systems Division, 1978.)

Figure 3–12. Generation of an output signal for a rotate-only CT system. (Courtesy of General Electric, Medical Systems Division, 1978.)

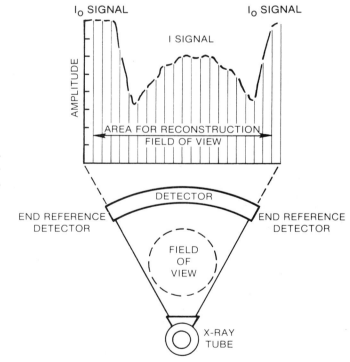

CT / 3

SUMMARY/REFERENCES/BIBLIOGRAPHY/REVIEW QUESTIONS

Summary

1. The x-ray source requirements in CT depend on the radiation attenuation and the intensity rate desired.

2. Clinical CT scanners use conventional x-ray sources, since they provide the greatest radiation intensity.

3. Two types of sources are used. These are fixed-anode oil-cooled tubes and rotating-anode air-cooled tubes, which can be pulsed in operation.

4. The purpose of a filter in CT is twofold. First, it increases beam quality (hardens beam) by absorbing low-energy waves, and, secondly, it can be shaped to provide uniform x-ray transmission.

5. The technique of collimation is important in CT, since it relates to patient dose and image quality. X-ray tube and detector collimation schemes are discussed. Several other important points on collimation are listed.

6. Some important findings of a study based on performance characteristics of collimators (Thomas et al., 1978) are presented.

7. Detectors used in CT are of two types. These are scintillation detectors and gas-ionization detectors. Several properties of detectors are given and discussed briefly.

8. A scintillation detector uses a scintillation crystal (e.g., NaI) coupled to a photomultiplier tube. The system converts radiation into electric current signals, which are fed into the computer for processing.

9. The gas ionization detector uses a pressurized gas chamber (e.g., xenon), which converts the radiation (passing through the patient) to electric current signals that are fed into the computer for processing.

10. The research findings of a split-detector system (Brooks and DiChiro, 1978) and the use of HgI_2 as CT detectors (Beinglass et al., 1980) are presented.

11. The electrical signals (analog information) received from the detectors are converted into digital information for computer reconstruction.

12. Finally, a comparison of the criteria for data acquisition and response time is given.

References

Beinglass, I., Kaufman, L., Hoisier, K., and Hoenninger, J.: An evaluation of HgI$_2$ detectors for x-ray computed tomography. Med. Phys., 7(4):370–373, 1980.

Brooks, R. A., and DiChiro, G.: Split-detector computed tomography — A preliminary report. Radiology, *126*:255–257, 1978.

Christensen, E. E., Curry, T. S., and Dowdey, J. E.: An Introduction to the Physics of Diagnostic Radiology, 2nd Ed. Philadelphia, Lea and Febiger, 1978, pp. 336–339.

General Electric Company: Facts about Xenon Detectors and GE Fast-scan Computed Tomography (Brochure). Milwaukee, Wisconsin, General Electric, Medical Systems Division, 1977.

General Electric Company: Personal communications with Medical Systems Division, 1978.

McCullough, E. C., and Payne, J. T.: X-ray transmission computed tomography. Med. Phys., 4(2):85–98, 1978.

Thomas, S. R., et al.: An evaluation of the performance characteristics of different types of collimators used with the EMI brain scanner (MK1) and their significance in specific clinical applications. Med. Phys., 5(2):124–132, 1978.

Bibliography

Brooks, R. A., and DiChiro, G.: Split-detector computed tomography — A preliminary report. Radiology, *126*:255–257, 1978.

Christensen, E. E., Curry, T. S., and Dowdey, J. E.: An Introduction to the Physics of Diagnostic Radiology, 2nd Ed. Philadelphia, Lea and Febiger, 1978, pp. 336–339.

Review Questions

1. In clinical CT, monochromatic sources of radiation are not used because:
   (a) They can produce problems related to shielding.
   (b) They have low radiation intensities.
   (c) They can create difficulties in equipment mechanics.
   (d) All of the above.

2. The most important reason for the use of conventional x-ray sources in CT is:
   (a) They have adequate shielding.
   (b) They have inherent filtration.
   (c) They are easily available.
   (d) Their radiation intensities are adequate to produce the transmission necessary in CT imaging.

3. The purpose of filtration in CT is:
   (a) To absorb "soft" radiation.
   (b) To increase beam quality.
   (c) To produce uniform x-ray transmission.
   (d) All of the above.

4. Which of the following determines the thickness of the section in CT?
   (a) The collimation of the x-ray beam
   (b) The pixel width
   (c) The computer program
   (d) The speed of rotation of the gantry

5. The purpose of a CT detector is:
   (a) To determine the number of slices to be obtained.
   (b) To measure the amount of scattered radiation.
   (c) To measure the x-ray transmission through the patient.
   (d) All of the above.

6. What property of a detector relates to the time for it to send out a signal and to recover so that it may send out another signal?
   (a) Stability
   (b) Response time
   (c) Uniformity
   (d) Quantum detection efficiency

7. Which of the following has *not* been used in a CT detection system?
   (a) Calcium fluoride
   (b) Cesium iodide
   (c) Calcium tungstate
   (d) Xenon gas

8. In which system is it possible to obtain two CT images at the same time?
   (a) The dual-energy method
   (b) The split-detector system
   (c) The translate/rotate system with one detector
   (d) One that uses two Polaroid cameras to record images

9. Which of the following CT detectors exhibits afterglow?
   (a) Xenon
   (b) Bismuth germanate
   (c) Calcium fluoride
   (d) Sodium iodide

10. Which of the following is true for scintillation CT detectors?
   (a) The amount of light produced in the crystals is directly proportional to the number of dynodes.
   (b) The amount of light produced in the crystals is directly proportional to the energy of the absorbed radiation.
   (c) The amount of light produced in the crystal is inversely proportional to the percentage of photons detected.
   (d) The amount of light produced in the crystals is not related to any property of the radiation beam.

CHAPTER 4

BASIC MATHEMATICAL CONCEPTS

The solutions to many problems in physics, and particularly medical physics, depend on being able to infer a density of matter in space from projections of the density onto planes.

A. M. CORMACK (1973)

Since the introduction of CT to clinical radiology, a number of articles on mathematical concepts of CT image reconstruction have appeared. As pointed out by Brooks and DiChiro (1975), these concepts are important to a basic understanding of the principles of CT.

It is essential for the reader to realize that CT has its roots in mathematical techniques, and therefore the concepts to be presented in this chapter will undoubtedly lead to a clearer comprehension of the basic problem to be solved. Just as Chapter 1 presented an overview of the computer necessary for an understanding of its application in CT, so it is the objective of this chapter to bring together the basic mathematics needed for a further insight into CT.

The descriptions of these mathematical approaches range from complex (Dehnert and Boyd, 1973; Sweeney and Vest, 1973; Herman and Rowland, 1973; Zwick and Zeitler, 1973; Gordon and Herman, 1974; Cho et al., 1975) to less rigorous treatments of the subject (Gordon et al., 1975; Edholm, 1975; Peters, 1975; Brooks and DiChiro, 1975) particularly intended for the clinically oriented community.

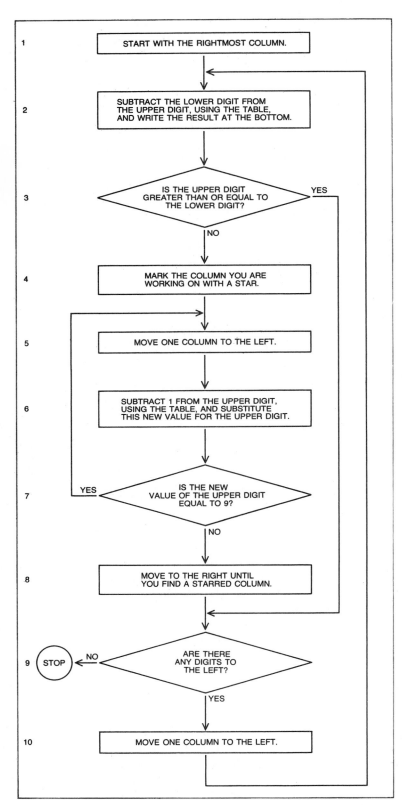

Figure 4–1. An example of an algorithm for the subtraction of whole numbers. (From Lewis, H.R., and Papadimitrion, C.H.: The Efficiency of Algorithms. Sci. Am., *238*:98, 1978. Reproduced by permission.)

ALGORITHM for the subtraction of whole numbers defines an explicit procedure that can be followed without any need for intuition and even without an understanding of the significance each step has to the operation as a whole. The algorithm, which is assumed to incorporate the table of differences shown here, can be applied to an infinite number of subtraction problems. Other algorithms are equally effective. A method of subtraction taught in European schools, for example, differs in the treatment of borrowing where it specifies that 1 should be added to the lower digit instead of being subtracted from the upper one.

The approaches utilize other basic mathematical concepts relating to logarithms, as well as solutions to simultaneous and integral equations. Since these concepts are probably not new (for the reader undoubtedly studied them in secondary school or college mathematics), they will not be treated in this chapter. However, two concepts that warrant brief consideration are algorithms and the Fourier transform, as these will aid tremendously in understanding the nature of image reconstruction.

ALGORITHMS

Today, the word *algorithm* has become very common, as a result of the impact of computer technology on everyday life. The word is derived from the Persian scholar Abu Ja' far Mohammed ibn Mûsâ alKowârîzmî, whose textbook on arithmetic (about A.D. 825) had a significant influence on mathematics for many years (Knuth, 1977). An algorithm is

> . . . a set of rules or directions for getting a specific output from a specific input. The distinguishing feature of an algorithm is that all vagueness must be eliminated; the rules must describe operations that are so simple and well defined, they can be executed by a machine. Furthermore, an algorithm must always terminate after a finite number of steps (Knuth, 1977).

In CT, the computer uses a suitable program to reconstruct the image. The type of program it uses is generally called an algorithm. A good example of an algorithm (Fig. 4–1) is the series of steps involved in the subtraction of whole numbers (Lewis and Papadimitrion, 1978). For the ambitious reader, a paper on computer algorithms for CT has been written by Cho and Ahn (1975).

FOURIER TRANSFORM

A radiologic image represents a variation of x-ray absorption coefficients, as shown in Figure 4–2. A plot of the distribution of coefficients as a function of

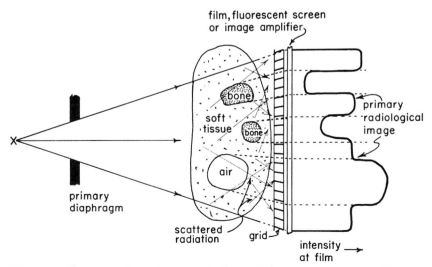

Figure 4–2. Formation of radiologic image through absorption and transmission of radiation. (From Johns, H.E., and Cunningham, J.R.: The Physics of Radiology, 3rd Ed. Springfield, IL, Charles C Thomas, 1969, p. 581. Reproduced by permission.)

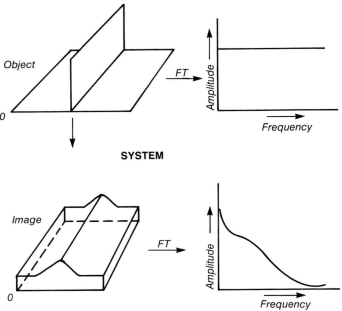

Figure 4–3. Simple illustration of the Fourier transform. (Adapted from Hay, G.A.: X-ray imaging. J. Phys. [E.], *11*:371–386, 1978, by permission.)

distance would generate a waveform of frequencies and amplitudes. This waveform can be approximated by a series of sine and cosine waves of different amplitudes and frequencies. To do this requires the use of the Fourier transform (FT).

In FT, the original waveform (image pattern) is resolved into sinusoidal components. The amplitudes are referred to as Fourier coefficients. By using these Fourier coefficients it is possible to reconstruct the original object pattern (McCullough and Payne, 1977). An illustration of the Fourier transform is shown in Figure 4–3. The use of Fourier transform techniques allows for faster, more accurate image reconstruction than do iterative mathematical techniques.

MATHEMATICAL TECHNIQUES

HISTORICAL OVERVIEW

Mathematical techniques using projections as a means of determining an object were first used in 1917 by Radon to solve gravitational problems. Within the past decades these methods have been used to solve other problems in astronomy and optics. It is not within the scope of this section to present an exhaustive account of historical notes; however, Figure 4–4 gives a brief summary of the development of image reconstruction mathematics and the areas to which they were first applied before utilization in CT.

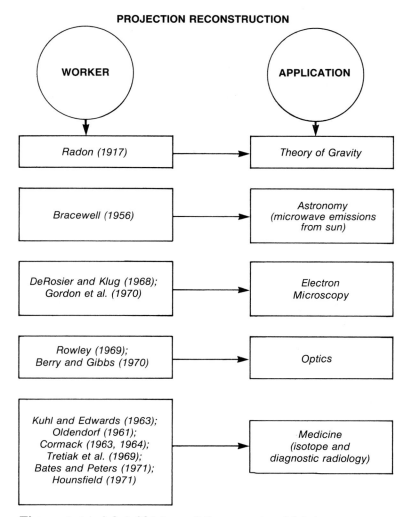

PROJECTION RECONSTRUCTION

WORKER

APPLICATION

| Radon (1917) | → | Theory of Gravity |

| Bracewell (1956) | → | Astronomy (microwave emissions from sun) |

| DeRosier and Klug (1968); Gordon et al. (1970) | → | Electron Microscopy |

| Rowley (1969); Berry and Gibbs (1970) | → | Optics |

| Kuhl and Edwards (1963); Oldendorf (1961); Cormack (1963, 1964); Tretiak et al. (1969); Bates and Peters (1971); Hounsfield (1971) | → | Medicine (isotope and diagnostic radiology) |

Figure 4–4. A brief history of the areas to which image reconstruction techniques were applied.

THE COMPUTATION PROBLEM

Consider Figure 4–5. In stating the problem in its most fundamental form, Cormack (1973) points out:

> . . . let O be the object in which there is a variable density, and P be the plane on which the density is projected. The object is thought of as being cut up into a number of slices, such as S, which project onto strips on P. The projection of the density in a cylinder C of S onto P yields the observed data. The problem is then idealized by allowing the thickness of the slice to vanish so that it becomes a plane, and the strip becomes a line, and simultaneously allowing the cylinder to shrink to a line. The value of the projected density at a point on P is the line integral of the density along the straight line through O. The mathematical problem is then to determine the density in the plane knowing the line integrals of the density along lines in the plane. It is clear that unless the object has some known symmetry (e.g., is spherically or cylindrically symmetrical) more than one projection will be needed, and an additional problem is to determine how many projections are needed to reconstruct the density to a prescribed degree of accuracy.

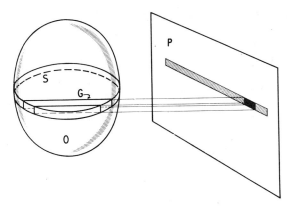

Figure 4–5. The expression of the computational problem in CT, in its most fundamental form. See text for explanation. (From Cormack, A.M.: Reconstruction of densities from their projections with applications in radiological physics. Phys. Med. Biol., *18*(2):195–207, 1973. Reproduced by permission.)

The same problem can be stated quantitatively. Consider an object O, represented by an x-y coordinate system, in Figure 4–6. The distribution of all attenuation coefficients (μ) is given by $\mu(x,y)$, which varies from point to point in the object. Suppose a pencil beam of x-rays of intensity I_0 from the x-ray source passes through the object along a straight path b, and the intensity of the emergent beam (falling on the CT detector) is I. Then a projection is given by the line integral of $\mu(x,y)$.

$$I = I_0 \exp \left[- \sum_{source}^{detector} \mu(x,y) \right]$$

By taking the negative logarithms, the above equation can be linearized to generate integral equations of the form

$$T_\theta(x) = \ln \left(\frac{I}{I_0} \right)$$

$$\ln \left(\frac{I_0}{I} \right) = \sum_{source}^{detector} \mu(x,y)$$

where $T_\theta(x)$ is the x-ray transmission at angle θ, which is really a measure of the total absorption along the straight line b (Fig. 4–6). $T_\theta(x)$ is referred to as the *ray sum* (Gordon and Herman, 1974). Stated in simple terms, the ray sum is the integral of $\mu(x,y)$ along the ray.

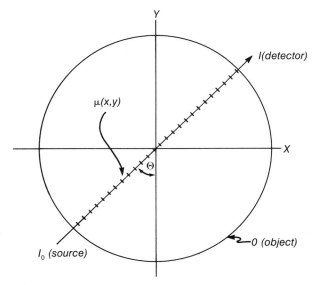

Figure 4–6. The total distribution of attenuation coefficients in object 0 is μ (x,y). The problem in CT is to calculate $\mu(x,y)$ from a set of projections specified by the angle θ. I_0 and I represent beam intensities from the source and at the detector, respectively.

The computational problem in CT, then, is to find $\mu(x,y)$ from the ray sums for a sufficiently large number of beams which passes through the object O. Hence, the scanning modes used in CT equipment (Chap. 2) ensure that every point in the object is scanned successively by a large set of transmission measurements (ray sums) $T_\theta(x)$.

COMPUTATIONAL METHODS

There are a number of computational methods available for calculating μ (x,y) from a set of projection data $T_\theta(x)$, but only those methods which have been used in clinical CT scanners will be discussed. The methods are shown in Figure 4–7 and follow a classification given by Brooks and DiChiro (1975).

Back Projection

Back projection is a simple procedure and does not require much mathematics to understand the concept. Back projection, also referred to as the

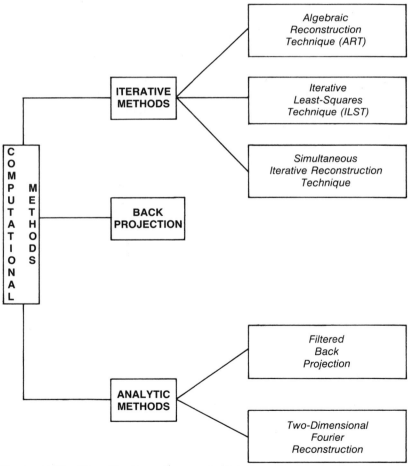

Figure 4–7. Classification of computational methods for CT. (Adapted from a table by Brooks, R.A., and DiChiro, G.: Principles of computer assisted tomography (CAT) in radiographic and radioisotopic imaging. Radiology, *117*:689–732, 1975. By permission.)

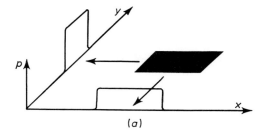

(a)

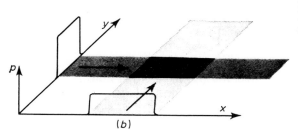

(b)

Figure 4–8. Graphical approach to the back projection reconstruction method. (From Brooks, R.A., and DiChiro, G.: Principles of computer assisted tomography (CAT) in radiographic and radioisotopic imaging. Phys. Med. Biol., *21*:698, 1976. By permission.)

summation method or the *linear superposition method,* was first used by Oldendorf (1961) and by Kuhl and Edwards (1963). Another approach used to describe back projection is the graphical method.

Consider two beams of x-rays passing through a rectangular object to produce two "penetration profiles," as shown in Figure 4–8*A*. The problem in CT is to reconstruct these profiles to give the original object. This is accomplished by back projecting the profiles (Fig. 4–8*B*), and the total distribution forms the CT image.

Back projection can also be explained by using the following numerical illustration (General Electric Company, 1976). Consider an object divided up into four squares (i.e., a 2 × 2 matrix with 4 pixels).

L		R
0	2
1	3

Initial Starting Point

a. Horizontal ray sum for top row is 2 (0+2).
b. Horizontal ray sum for bottom row is 4 (1+3).
c. Vertical ray sum for column to the left is 1 (0+1).
d. Vertical ray sum for column to the right is 5 (2+3).
e. Right diagonal ray sums are 0, 3 (2+1), and 3.
f. Left diagonal ray sums are 1, 3 (0+3), and 2.

2	2
4	4

1st Guess

Place horizontal ray sums from the previous 2 × 2 matrix (i.e., 2 and 4) in each of the squares to obtain the first guess.

3	7
5	9

2nd Guess

Add the vertical ray sums from the original 2 × 2 matrix (i.e., 1 and 5) to the value in each of the squares in the first guess; that is

$$1 + 2 = 3$$
$$1 + 4 = 5$$
$$5 + 2 = 7$$
$$5 + 4 = 9$$

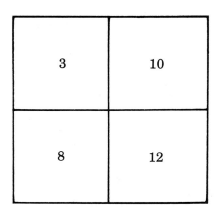

3rd Guess

Add the diagonal ray sums (right) from the original 2 × 2 matrix to the values in the second guess; that is

$$0 + 3 = 3$$
$$3 + 5 = 8$$
$$3 + 7 = 10$$
$$3 + 9 = 12$$

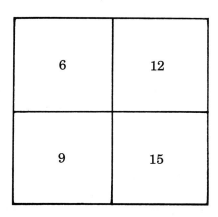

4th Guess

Add the diagonal ray sums (left) from the original 2 × 2 matrix to the values in the third guess; that is

$$3 + 3 = 6$$
$$2 + 10 = 12$$
$$3 + 12 = 15$$
$$1 + 8 = 9$$

The next step is to obtain the original matrix. This can be done as follows:

a. Subtract the *constant value,* 6, from each square in the fourth guess. This gives

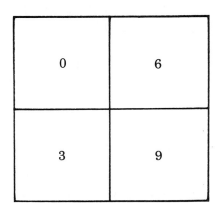

b. Now, the problem is to reduce the preceding matrix to a simple ratio. Hence, by using the obvious common divisor, 3, the following is obtained:

0	2
1	3

This is the original 2 × 2 matrix.

One of the fundamental limitations of back projection is that it does not produce a sharply defined image of the original object, and it requires substantial computation time. Hence, the use of this method in CT has been discontinued, since it does not meet present-day clinical resolution requirements. The "most striking artifact" of this technique is that of the classical star pattern, which occurs because points outside a high-density object receive some of the back-projected intensity of that object (Brooks and DiChiro, 1975).

Iterative Methods

Another common method of reconstruction is based on iterative techniques. *Iterative* is a term used to refer to a "method of successive approximations in which an arbitrary starting image is chosen, corrections are applied to bring it into better agreement with the measured projections and then new corrections are applied, etc., until satisfactory agreement is obtained" (Brooks and DiChiro, 1975).

Several techniques have been discussed by Brooks and DiChiro (1975) and by Gordon and Herman (1974). These include (a) simultaneous iterative reconstruction technique (SIRT), (b) iterative least-squares technique (ILST), and (c) algebraic reconstruction technique (ART). These techniques differ in the way corrections are applied to subsequent iterations. In this section only the ART method will be considered.

The ART was used by Hounsfield in the first EMI brain scanner (Hounsfield, 1972). For the sake of simplicity, consider the following numerical illustration:

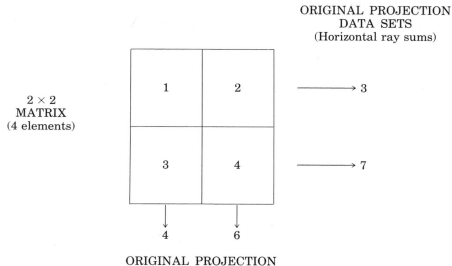

ORIGINAL PROJECTION
DATA SETS
(Horizontal ray sums)

2 × 2
MATRIX
(4 elements)

ORIGINAL PROJECTION
DATA SETS
(Vertical ray sums)

NEW PROJECTION
DATA SETS
(Horizontal ray sums)

a. INITIAL ESTIMATE
Compute average of
4 elements and
assign to each
pixel; that is,
$1 + 2 + 3 + 4 = 10$
$10 \div 4 = 2.5$

2.5	2.5
2.5	2.5

⟶ 5

⟶ 5

b. FIRST CORREC-
TION FOR ERROR
(Original horizontal
ray sums minus the
new horizontal ray
sums divided by 2)
$= \dfrac{3-5}{2}$ and $\dfrac{7-5}{2}$

$= \dfrac{-2}{2}$ and $\dfrac{2}{2}$

$= -1.0$ and 1.0

$(2.5 - 1.0)$ 1.5	$(2.5 - 1.0)$ 1.5
$(2.5 + 1.0)$ 3.5	$(2.5 + 1.0)$ 3.5

c. SECOND ESTIMATE

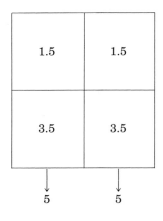

| 1.5 | 1.5 |
| 3.5 | 3.5 |

↓   ↓
5   5

NEW PROJECTION
DATA SETS
(Vertical ray sums)

d. SECOND CORREC-
TION FOR ERROR
(Original vertical
ray sums minus
new vertical ray
sums divided by 2)

$$= \frac{4-5}{2} \text{ and } \frac{6-5}{2}$$

$$= \frac{-1.0}{2} \text{ and } \frac{+1.0}{2}$$

$$= -0.5 \text{ and } +0.5$$

| (1.5 − 0.5)   1 | (1.5 + 0.5)   2 |
| (3.5 − 0.5)   3 | (3.5 + 0.5)   4 |

The final matrix solution is thus

| 1 | 2 |
| 3 | 4 |

Today these techniques are not used in commercial scanners because of the following limitations:

1. It is difficult to obtain accurately measured ray sums due to quantum noise and patient motion.

2. The procedure takes too long to generate the reconstructed image, since the iteration can be done only when all projection data sets are obtained.

3. In order to produce a "true" image there should be more projection data sets (ray sums) than pixels. (Therefore, diagonal projection data sets are taken to eliminate ambiguity.)

ANALYTIC RECONSTRUCTION TECHNIQUES

Analytic reconstruction techniques can also be used to reconstruct images from their projections. These methods have sound mathematical bases (not within the scope of this text) and are used in most commercial CT scanners today. Essentially they are (a) the Fourier method and (b) filtered back projection or convolution method.

Both methods are faster than iterative methods and yield accurate results.

The Fourier Method

The Fourier method is also referred to as two-dimensional Fourier reconstruction. Recall the section on Fourier transformation. In brief, it states that any function can be broken down mathematically into a number of frequencies and amplitudes and that the amplitudes are referred to as Fourier coefficients. In order to understand the method, consider the following example given by Brooks and DiChiro (1975). Incoming sound waves to the ear can be separated out into different signals with different intensity levels (Fourier components). The signals then arrive at the brain, which rearranges them to produce a perception of the original sound.

In the Fourier method of reconstruction, the same principle applies. In general if the Fourier coefficients of the projections are known, then an image of the object can be reconstructed.

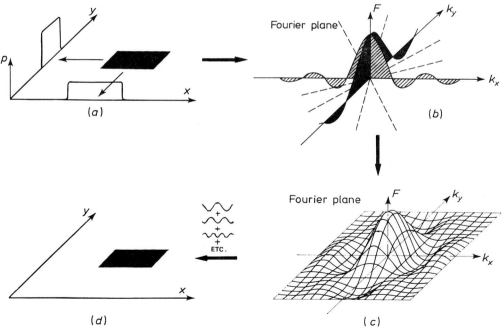

Figure 4–9. Illustration of the Fourier method of image reconstruction. (From Brooks, R.A., and DiChiro, G.: Principles of computer assisted tomography (CAT) in radiographic and radioisotopic imaging. Phys. Med. Biol., *21*:709, 1976. Reproduced by permission.)

The Fourier method is illustrated in Figure 4–9 and consists of the following operations:

a. Projections are obtained by irradiating the object (rectangle). In this case only two projections are shown (Fig. 4–9A).

b. Fourier coefficents are obtained from the projections and are "plotted at corresponding angles in the Fourier plane" (Fig. 4–9B).

c. These coefficients are used to form a rectangular array using interpolation techniques (Bracewell, 1965) (Fig. 4–9C).

d. In the final stages, the image is reconstructed by summing the Fourier coefficients (i.e., adding the waveforms) (Fig. 4–9D).

Filtered Back Projection

Filtered back projection is also known as the *convolution method*. It is similar to that of back projection. In this method, all projection data are filtered or convolved (using suitable filtering formulas) before they are back projected, to produce an image free of streak artifacts. These formulas are mathematically rigorous and for this reason will not be treated here.

Recall that in the back projection method image sharpness is reduced by a "starlike" blurring pattern. In filtered back projection, this blurring is eliminated. Again, it is done by using suitable filtering formulas (correction functions). Figure 4–10 illustrates the concept of convolution in simple terms. Briefly,

a. All projection data sets are obtained.

b. The logarithm of each data point is obtained.

c. The logarithmic values are multiplied by a convolution filter formula and the filtered values are then back projected.

d. In the final stages, i.e., in summing the filtered projections, the negative and positive components cancel each other out, thus producing an image free of blurring.

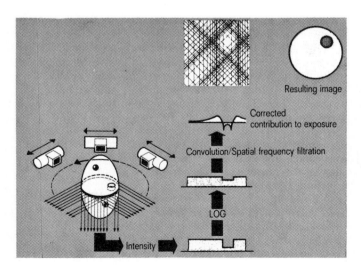

Figure 4–10. The convolution technique. See text for explanation. (From Pfeiler, M., Schwierz, G., and Linke, G.: Some guiding ideas on imaging recording in computerized axial tomography. Electromedica, *1*:19–25, 1976. Reproduced by permission.)

COMPARISON OF RECONSTRUCTION METHODS

A comparison of the various methods of image reconstruction can be very lengthy and mathematically rigorous (Cho et al., 1975; Dehnert and Boyd, 1973). Such comparison is beyond the scope of this section; however, the interested reader can refer to the paper by Brooks and DiChiro (1975). The following is a brief summary of their discussion with respect to speed, accuracy, and versatility:

Speed. Analytic methods are faster than iterative methods. Image reconstruction time is a function of several factors, including "the size of the image and the number of projections" (Brooks and DiChiro, 1975).

Accuracy. Analytic methods may generate very accurate results faster than iterative methods, depending on factors relating to the data.

Versatility. Iterative methods yield "better performance in some situations with incomplete data" (Brooks and DiChiro, 1975). Iterative methods are more versatile. Both methods can be used in scanners using fan-beam geometry (Brooks and DiChiro, 1975).

CT / 4

SUMMARY/REFERENCES/BIBLIOGRAPHY/REVIEW QUESTIONS

Summary

1. In this chapter, mathematical methods for image reconstruction from projections are presented briefly, without resorting to the use of rigorous mathematics.

2. The concepts of an algorithm (a set of rules for solving a problem in a specified number of steps) and the Fourier transform are given, as these are necessary to a further understanding of CT mathematics.

3. The history of these mathematical techniques dates back to 1917. A brief summary is given in Figure 4-4.

4. The problem in CT is to calculate all attenuation coefficients represented in the object, knowing a large number of x-ray transmission measurements.

5. The concept of ray sum is pointed out. This is really a transmission measurement along a ray at a given angle.

6. Computational methods in CT are back projection, iterative methods, and analytic methods.

7. Back projection was used in earlier studies. It involves obtaining profiles of an object and then back projecting them. The total distribution forms the CT image. A numerical illustration was used to further elucidate back projection.

8. Iterative methods were used by Hounsfield in the first EMI scanner. This kind of reconstruction involves choosing a starting image (guess) and applying a series of repetitive operations in which corrections are used to produce an image of the original object. A numerical illustration was used to describe the method.

9. Analytical techniques are of two types, the Fourier method and the convolution or filtered back projection method. These methods are mathematically rigorous, and hence they were described only briefly. The methods are used in most commercial scanners.

10. The Fourier method is based on Fourier transformation. Using Fourier coefficients (amplitudes) of the projections, an image of the object can be reconstructed.

11. The convolution method, on the other hand, is similar to back projection. Here, the projection data are filtered or convolved before they are back projected to produce a sharper image than the one obtained by the simple back projection technique.

12. Finally, a comparison of reconstruction methods is given with respect to speed, accuracy, and versatility.

References

Bracewell, R. N.: The Fourier Transform and its Applications. New York, McGraw-Hill Book Co., 1965.

Brooks, R. A., and DiChiro, G.: Theory of image reconstruction in computed tomography. Radiology, *117*:561–572, 1975.

Brooks, R. A., and DiChiro, G.: Principles of computer assisted tomography (CAT) in radiographic and radioisotopic imaging. Phys. Med. Biol., *21*(5):689–732, 1976.

Cho, Z. H., and Ahn, I. S.: Computer algorithms for the tomographic image reconstruction with x-ray transmission scans. Comput. Biomed. Res., *8*:8–25, 1975.

Cho, Z. H., Chan, J. K., Hall, E. L., et al.: A comparative study of 3-D image reconstruction algorithms and noise filtering. IEEE Trans. Nucl. Sci., *NS-22*(1):344–358, 1975.

Cormack, A. M.: Reconstruction of densities from their projections with applications in radiological physics. Phys. Med. Biol., *18*(2):195–207, 1973.

Dehnert, J., and Boyd, G.: A comparison study of some computer reconstruction techniques. High Energy Physics. Lab. Rep. 276. Stanford University, California, July, 1973.

Edholm, P.: Image construction in transversal computer tomography. Acta Radiol. (Suppl.), *346*:21–38, 1975.

General Electric Company: Introduction to Computed Tomography. Milwaukee, Wisconsin, General Electric Company, Medical Systems Division, 1976.

Gordon, R., and Herman, G. T.: Three-dimensional reconstruction from projections. A review of algorithms. Int. Rev. Cytol., *38*:111, 1974.

Gordon, R., Herman, G. T., and Johnson, S. A.: Image reconstruction from projections. Sci. Am., *233*:56–61, 64–68, 1975.

Hay, G. A.: X-ray imaging. J. Phys. [E], *11*:377–386, 1978.

Herman, G. T., and Rowland, S.: Three methods for reconstructing objects from x-rays. A comparative study. Comput. Graph. Image Process., *2*:151–178, 1973.

Hounsfield, G. N.: A method of and apparatus for examination of a body by radiation such as x- or gamma radiation. British Patent No. 1283915. London, 1972.

Johns, H. E., and Cunningham, J. R.: The Physics of Radiology. Springfield, Ill., Charles C Thomas, Publisher, 1969.

Knuth, D. E.: Algorithms. Sci. Am. *236*:63–80, 1977.

Kuhl, D. E., and Edwards, R. Q.: Image separation radioisotope scanning. Radiology, *80*:653–661, 1963.
Lewis, H. R., and Papadimitrion, C. H.: The efficiency of algorithms. Sci. Am., *238*:96–109, 1978.
McCullough, E. C., and Payne, J. T.: X-ray transmission computed tomography. Med. Phys., *4*(2):85–98, 1977.
Oldendorf, W. H.: Isolated flying spot detection of radiodensity discontinuities displaying the internal structural pattern of a complex object. IRE Trans. Biomed. Elect., *BME8:*68–72, 1961.
Peters, T. M.: Principles of computerized tomography. Australas. Radiol., *19*:118–126, 1975.
Pfeiler, M., Schwierz, G., and Linke, G.: Some guiding ideas on image recording in computerized axial tomography. Electromedica, *1*:19–25, 1976.
Sweeney, D. W., and Vest, C. M.: Reconstruction of three-dimensional refractive index fields from multidirectional interferometric data. Appl. Optics, *12*:2649–2664, 1973.
Zwick, M., and Zeitler, E.: Image reconstruction from projections. Optik, *38*:550–565, 1973.

Bibliography

Gordon, R., Herman, G. T., and Johnson, S. A.: Image reconstruction from projections. Sci. Am., *233*:56–61, 64–68, 1975.
Knuth, D. E.: Algorithms. Sci. Am., *236*:63–80, 1977.
Pfeiler, M., Schwierz, G., and Linke, G.: Some guiding ideas on image recording in computerized axial tomography. Electromedica, *1*:19–25, 1976.
Pullan, B. R.: Computerized axial tomography. Phys. Educ., *13*:92–96, 1978.

Review Questions

1. Which of the following describes a set of rules for solving a problem using a specified number of steps?
    (a) Algorithm
    (b) Logarithm
    (c) Fourier transform
    (d) Attenuation coefficient

2. The first reconstruction from projections was used by
    (a) Radon.
    (b) Hounsfield.
    (c) Roentgen.
    (d) Kuhl.

3. Image reconstruction techniques were used earlier to solve problems in:
    (a) Optics and electron microscopy.
    (b) Gravity.
    (c) Astronomy.
    (d) All of the above.

4. Who applied reconstruction techniques to solve problems in the theory of gravity?
    (a) Radon
    (b) Hounsfield
    (c) Roentgen
    (d) Rowley

5. Which of the following is *not* an iterative method of image reconstruction from projections?
    (a) Algebraic reconstruction technique
    (b) Simultaneous iterative reconstructive technique
    (c) Iterative least-squares technique
    (d) Two-dimensional Fourier reconstruction

6. Which of the following involves applying suitable filtering formulas to the projection data before they are back projected to produce an image free of blurring?
   (a) Back projection
   (b) Iterative method
   (c) Fourier method
   (d) Convolution method

7. In which of the following is a *blurring* pattern present?
   (a) Back projection
   (b) Iterative method
   (c) Fourier method
   (d) Convolution method

8. With respect to accuracy, which of the following yields accurate results very quickly?
   (a) Algebraic reconstruction technique
   (b) Back projection
   (c) Convolution method
   (d) Iterative least-squares technique

9. The computational problem in CT is:
   (a) To compute all attenuation coefficients for soft tissues and bone, knowing the thickness of each slice.
   (b) To compute all attenuation coefficients, using only 50 x-ray transmission measurements.
   (c) To compute all attenuation coefficients in an object, using a large number of transmission readings.
   (d) To find out how many transmission readings are necessary to compute attenuation values.

10. Which of the following was used by Hounsfield in the first EMI brain scanner?
    (a) Convolution technique
    (b) Iterative technique
    (c) Back projection
    (d) Fourier technique

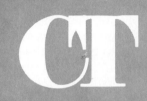

CHAPTER 5

EQUIPMENT

The first practical experiments of this new technique were carried out on a device constructed from an old metal-working lathe salvaged from EMI's mechanical engineering workshop.

EMI CENTRAL RESEARCH LABS (1977)

The rapid change in and development of CT techniques have made available a vast number of machines to scan the patient. Major improvements in engineering design and construction have resulted in a number of different prototypes available from several manufacturers of CT equipment (see Appendix A, p. 121).

A discussion of equipment characteristics is essential, since the radiologist, technologist, and others concerned are in direct control of a number of parameters that influence workload, patient care, and the acquisition of good diagnostic images. In this chapter, a number of basic elements fundamental to a total CT scanning system will be identified and discussed. The discussion is

89

intended to familiarize the reader with CT equipment through identification of the main components, since it would be fruitless to present details of each prototype commercially available. The chapter also introduces some associated terminology.

BASIC EQUIPMENT CONFIGURATION

The configuration to be used here represents a common scheme typical of "generations" of CT equipment. There are three major component systems. Figure 5–1 shows the main elements of these systems, which include (a) the imaging system (data acquisition), (b) the computer system (data manipulation), and (c) the image display and recording system.

THE IMAGING SYSTEM

Figure 5–2 shows the very first imaging system, which was used by Hounsfield in his original CT experiments. Today, similar components are still used with additional refinements. These are the x-ray generator, the x-ray tube, and the detector system. Another component that can be included here is

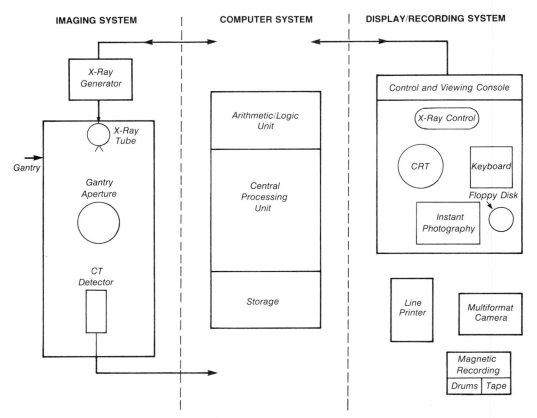

Figure 5–1. Basic configuration of a typical CT scanning system. The arrows indicate feedback and control among the three systems.

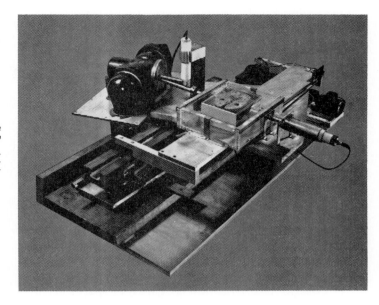

Figure 5–2. The original lathe bed scanner used in early CT experiments by G. N. Hounsfield of EMI. (Courtesy of EMI Medical, Inc.)

the patient's couch, although it does not play a fundamental role in data acquisition.

The x-ray generator need not be presented here, since most readers are familiar with basic principles of x-ray generation. The components that would be included here are those of the high-voltage transformer, the rectification circuits, the x-ray tube, the control unit, and sometimes other components as well.

The x-ray tube and detectors are housed in what is referred to as the *scanning gantry*. The gantry is really a framework mounted so that it surrounds the patient in a vertical plane. The gantry *aperture size* (an opening through which the patient moves during scanning) usually varies from system to system, typical aperture sizes varying from 45 to 66 cm.

The gantry can be made to tilt from the vertical position to allow for examination of specific structures in the patient. The degree of tilt will vary from system to system, but typical degrees of tilt are ±15 to 20° from the vertical position.

The couch provides a platform to hold the patient. The top is motorized and can be moved further through the aperture after each slice. This can be done automatically via the computer or manually by the operator. Additional controls allow for adjustments of table height, tilt, speed of travel, and so on.

In Figure 5–3, front views of four gantry types with patient couches are shown, while Figure 5–4 demonstrates a rear view of one gantry. In Figure 5–5 one can see how the detectors and x-ray tube are mounted in the gantry (fourth-generation system).

Positioning of the patient is aided by light beam indicators usually mounted on the gantry. This ensures speed and accuracy in positioning. One such system is shown in Figure 5–6. In some scanners laser beams are used to indicate the slice position. In this case, the patient should be instructed not to look into the laser beam, as this can be hazardous to the eyes. A warning of this sort should be provided by manufacturers of CT systems using laser beams for patient positioning.

Text continued on page 95

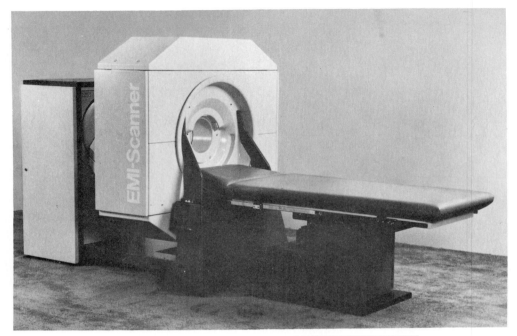

A

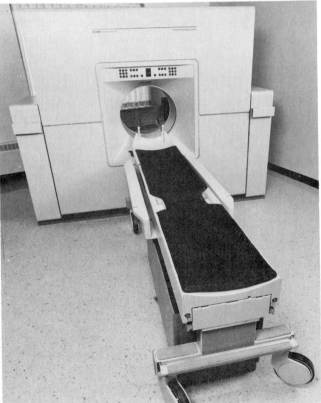

B

Figure 5–3.   Four different types of gantry systems with patient couches. (*A* courtesy of EMI Medical, Inc.; *B* courtesy of Picker International; *C* courtesy of Pfizer/American Science and Engineering; *D* courtesy of EMI Medical, Inc.)
Figure continued on opposite page

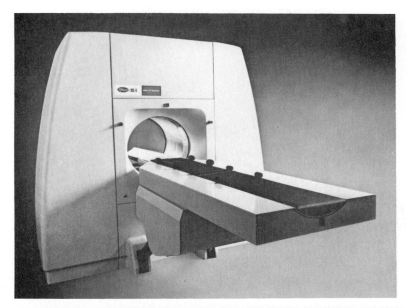

C

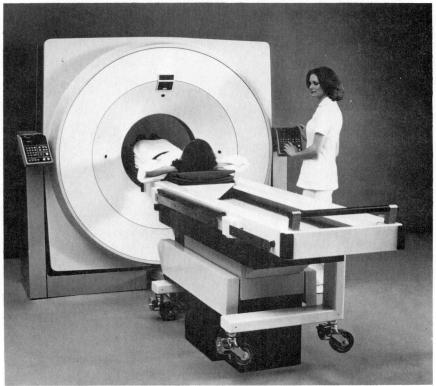

D

Figure 5–3 *Continued*

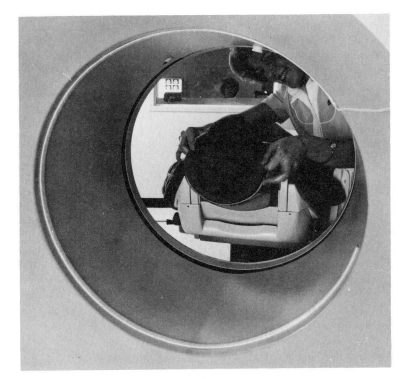

Figure 5-4. View behind aperture of one gantry system. (Courtesy of Picker International.)

Figure 5-5. Gantry system showing how detectors (outer circle) and x-ray tube (partially shown) are mounted ("fourth-generation"). (Courtesy of Pfizer/American Science and Engineering.)

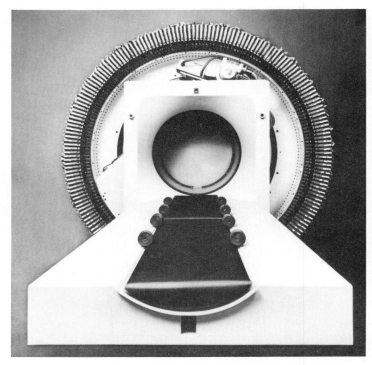

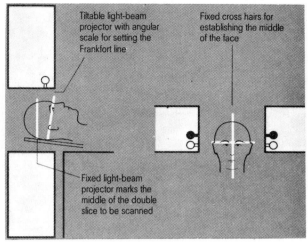

Tiltable light-beam projector with angular scale for setting the Frankfort line

Fixed cross hairs for establishing the middle of the face

Fixed light-beam projector marks the middle of the double slice to be scanned

Figure 5–6. The position of light-beam indicators for the SIRETOM 2000 (a Siemens CT unit) which aids in patient positioning. (From Krumme, H. J.: A new computerized tomographic head unit. The Siretom 2000. Electromedica 3-4:123–128, 1977. Reproduced by permission.)

THE COMPUTER SYSTEM

The information from the detectors (analog information) is converted into digital form and sent to the computer for processing. The computer is used to perform the following tasks (Krumme, 1977):

1. Communicates with the user with regard to data administration and dialogue.
2. Assists in technical maintenance (runs the gantry).
3. Directs and keeps track of radiation measurements.
4. Provides reconstruction and supplementary image processing.

The components of the computer system that would handle the above tasks are the central processing unit (CPU) and the input-output devices.

The Central Processing Unit (CPU)

The basic organization of the CPU and its function were already described in Chapter 1.

Storage in CT is facilitated by magnetic disks and magnetic tape. The image storage capacity for both will differ from system to system. For example, the image storage capacity of the main disk of the EMI Scanner 7070 is 192 Mbytes (1000 320 × 320 pictures), while for the dual floppy disk, it is 6 320 × 320 pictures per disk and 22 160 × 160 pictures per disk (EMI Medical, Inc., 1978).

The other important element of storage is the number of images that can be put on the tape. Again, this number will vary from system to system and will depend on reel size. The 267 mm. (10.5 in.) reel of the EMI 7070 scanner will hold 400 160 × 160 images or 250 320 × 320 (EMI Medical, Inc., 1978).

In Figure 5–7 CPU's and magnetic tape units for two CT systems are shown.

Most present-day computer systems in CT allow for *real time processing* by utilizing high-speed hardware processors. This means that the image can be displayed for viewing as scanning is in progress.

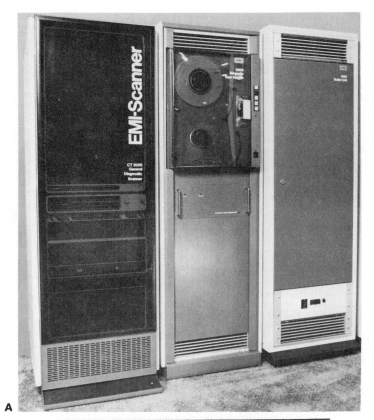

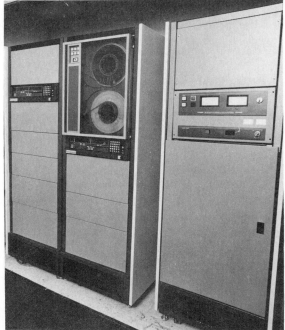

Figure 5–7.   Magnetic tape and central processing units for two CT systems. (*A* courtesy of EMI Medical, Inc.; *B* courtesy of Picker International.)

Input-Output Devices

Input-output devices include television monitors (CRT display), line printers, teletypes, etc. Recall from Chapter 1 that a CRT device with a keyboard can be used as an output device as well as an input device. These will be discussed in later sections.

IMAGE DISPLAY

After the computer processes the information, the reconstructed image must be displayed for viewing and recording.

The equipment for image display and documentation can include several consoles. One such console is the *control and viewing console* (operator's console), at which several functions can be performed. It is not possible to give complete descriptions of consoles, since individual consoles will differ from scanner to scanner. However, the important and more common features of a CT operator's console will be presented in a later section.

IMAGE DOCUMENTATION

Image documentation in CT refers to methods available to record and store the CT image. Commonly used documentation modes are film documentation and magnetic storage (tape or disks).

FILM DOCUMENTATION

Film documentation refers to the techniques of *instant-picture photography* (Polaroid camera and film) and *transparency* film. In the latter, this is achieved through the use of photographic recording on x-ray film (multi-image, multi-format camera). In this case, a number of different film formats is available, such as 70 mm., 90 mm., 100 mm., and 105 mm., 8 × 10 inch, 11 × 14 inch, and 14 × 17 inch, on which a number of images can be recorded per film sheet.

Since instant photography offers only a limited number of gray shades (8 to 10; although more shades are possible with newer films), transparency film is often used. With transparency film more shades of gray (16 to 20) and a higher definition can be perceived by the observer (Weckesser et al., 1978).

Additional image documentation in CT is also available, including the *hard-copy print-out* (numerical print-out — recall Chapter 2) and a print-out of *isodensity lines,* seen in Figure 5–8.

MAGNETIC STORAGE

Magnetic data carriers include magnetic tapes, magnetic disks, and floppy diskettes. These were already described in Chapter 1.

Magnetic tapes have greater storage capacity than disks and are advan-

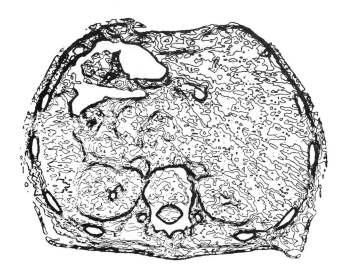

Figure 5–8. Hard-copy print-out of isodensity lines. (From Weckesser, W. D., Scharl, P., and Krumme, H. J.: CT image documentation — State of the art and outlook. Electromedica, *4*:122–127, 1978. Reproduced by permission.)

tageous for long-term storage. Other advantages together with disadvantages of tapes and floppy diskettes are given in Table 5–1.

A TECHNICAL NOTE

It was pointed out by Winter (1978) that artifacts may appear on CT photographic images due to nonsynchronization between the camera exposure and the television sweep. These artifacts include the appearance of dark and bright bands on the recorded image for camera exposure times shorter than 1/30 sec. and longer than 1/30 sec., respectively. The dark bands are due to the exclusion of "every other scan line over part of the picture," while bright bands "duplicate every other scan line over part of the picture" (Winter, 1978).

Winter (1978) suggests that "artifact-free" and sharper images can be obtained either by using synchronized cameras or by increasing exposure times, using smaller f-numbers and decreasing the brightness of the television picture tube.

TABLE 5–1.   ADVANTAGES AND DISADVANTAGES OF TWO DATA CARRIERS USED IN CT

DATA CARRIER	ADVANTAGES	DISADVANTAGES
Floppy diskette	Shorter access time. Easy to handle. Low "maintenance costs of drive mechanism." Can be included in patient's film envelope.	High cost
Magnetic tape	Inexpensive. Easily adaptable to other computer systems.	High costs for maintenance of drive mechanism. Long time to retrieve stored images. Sensitive to environmental changes.

After Weckesser, W. D., Scharl, P., and Krumme, H. J.: CT image documentation — State of the art and outlook. Electromedica, *4*:122–127, 1978.

THE CONTROL CONSOLE

CHARACTERISTIC FEATURES

The console in Figure 5–9 contains a number of features that are common to most CT control and viewing consoles.

Control Panel.   The panel usually displays the on-off switch for energizing the console, mA and kVp settings (x-ray factors), slice position, and push buttons to reset, abort, and commence scanning. A number of other buttons are available on the various models of CT equipment. Figure 5–10 shows a close-up view of a control panel.

Alphanumeric Keyboard.   Figure 5–10 shows an alphanumeric keyboard, which looks like a typewriter keyboard and contains both alphabetic characters (letters) and numeric characters (digits). The operator uses this keyboard to enter (input) information into the computer concerning the scanning procedure and other related information, such as patient's name, age, and sex. The number of keys and the functions denoted by some of them will differ from scanner to scanner and will be found in the appropriate equipment manuals.

CRT Display Device.   Figures 5–11 and 5–12 show CRT display devices. These are used to display the reconstructed image and a number of other parameters, including "contrast" settings, CT numbers, and the gray scale, age, weight, height, sex, number of the patient, slice number and location, and type and amount of contrast used.

Photographic Recording Equipment.   Most scanners are equipped with a camera coupled to a photographic monitor. From this monitor the operator records the images onto photographic film. Multi-image x-ray film cameras

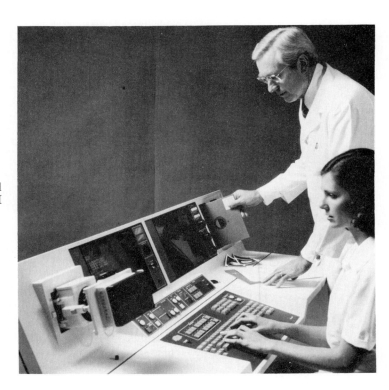

Figure 5–9.   A CT control console. (Courtesy of EMI Medical, Inc.)

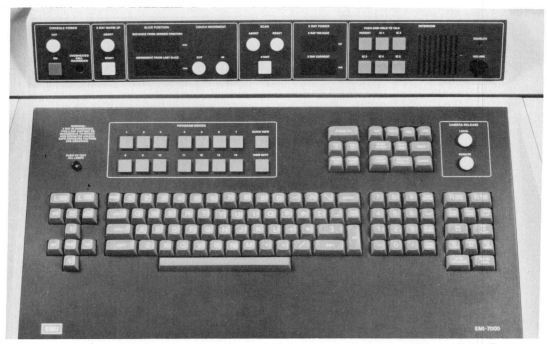

Figure 5–10. Close-up view of control panel of the same unit shown in Figure 5–9. (Courtesy of EMI Medical, Inc.)

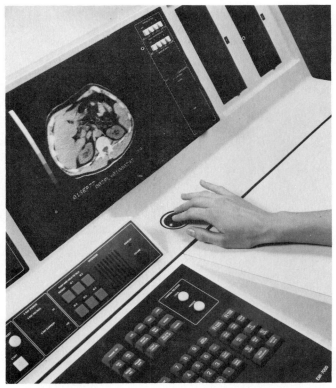

Figure 5–11. CRT display device for the EMI 7000 CT scanner. (Courtesy of EMI Medical, Inc.)

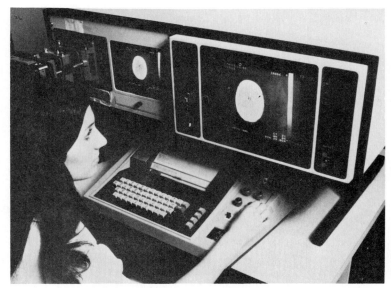

Figure 5–12.   CRT display device for an Ohio-Nuclear CT Scanner (Delta-Scan). (Courtesy of Ohio-Nuclear, Inc.)

(multi-imager) for transparent film are also used. Photographic equipment is shown in Figures 5–9 (lower left corner) and 5–12 (upper left corner).

Floppy Disk Drive.   In Figure 5–9 the man is inserting a disk into the drive mechanism for recording the CT image. A close-up of two drives is shown in Figure 5–11 (upper right corner).

Interactive Function Keys.   There are operational keys on the console other than the alphanumeric keys. The function and labeling of each key will differ from scanner to scanner. These function keys for one CT system are shown in Figure 5–13. The explanation of each key will not be given here, since this can be found in the equipment manual; however, the effects of two keys (edit data page and zoom) are shown in Figure 5–14.

Other function keys available on some scanners (e.g., EMI 6000 series) are the region of interest (ROI), highlight, point-to-point, and preview scan localization. These are illustrated and further explained in Figure 5–15. It is important to realize that other terms may be used (on different scanners) to achieve the same purpose as the keys just mentioned.

Other Controls.   There are a number of other controls available on CT control consoles. The two common ones that deserve mention here are the joystick and the trackball.

The *joystick* (a lever-type device) positions the region-of-interest rectangle (Fig. 5–15A) over any part of the CT image, which allows for further tissue density analysis. The joystick is the device that the operator in Figure 5–16 (shown in background) is touching.

The *trackball,* the device that the operator is touching in Figure 5–11, is used for the same purpose as the joystick. Some scanners have joysticks, while others have trackballs.

Window Width and Window Level Controls.   These are shown in Figure 5–11 and will be discussed later in the chapter under a separate section.

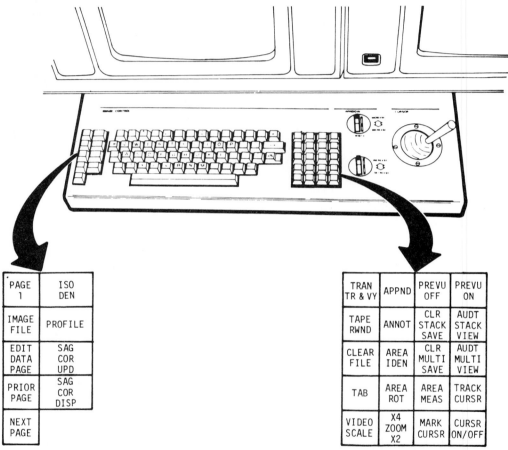

Figure 5–13.   Interactive function keys on console of the SYNERVIEW CT system. (Courtesy of Picker International.)

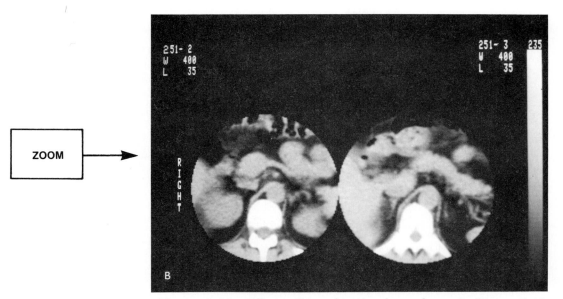

Figure 5–14. Effects of two function keys shown in Figure 5–13. (Photographs courtesy of Picker International.)

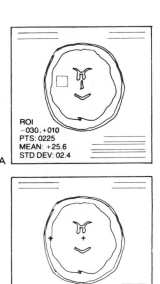

Region-of-Interest Mode

The ROI, controlled by a joy stick, permits the diagnostician to more thoroughly interrogate scan data.
Annotation includes:
a. Coordinates of ROI center
b. No. of points in ROI
c. Mean CT number
d. Standard deviation

ROI
−030,+010
PTS: 0225
MEAN: +25.6
STD DEV: 02.4

A

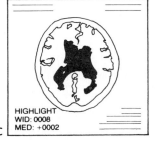

Point-to-Point

This mode permits the diagnostician to accurately measure the distance between any two points on the CRT.
Annotation specifies the distance between the two points in centimeters to one decimal place.

POINT TO POINT
DIST: 6.7 CM

B

Highlight

Highlight mode accentuates a range of CT numbers by driving them to end-level white or black. This is useful for readily identifying all tissue of similar densities.
Annotation includes:
a. Width of the highlight window
b. Median of the highlight window

HIGHLIGHT
WID: 0008
MED: +0002

C

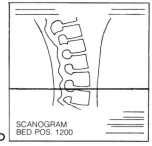

**Preview Scan Localization
(Scanogram)**

Lateral and PA projections enable accurate, computer-controlled couch/slice plane positioning via the Joy-stick controlled moveable cursor and the image annotation which specifies the corresponding bed position.

SCANOGRAM
BED POS. 1200

D

Figure 5–15. Diagrammatic representation of the effects of four function keys for one CT system. (Courtesy of EMI Medical, Inc.)

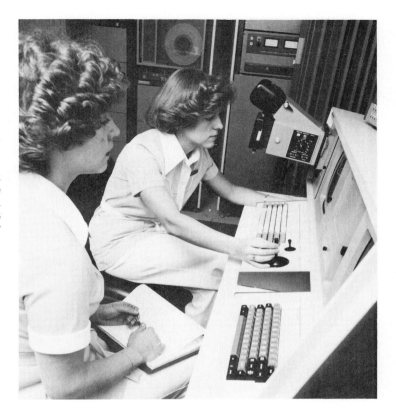

Figure 5–16. The joystick control (the device that the technologist in the background is touching with her right hand). (Courtesy of Picker International.)

OPTIONAL EQUIPMENT

Several optional pieces of equipment are available to add to a basic CT system with standard components. The more common ones are the line printer, the multi-image multi-format camera, and the physician- or diagnostic-viewing console. This console facilitates viewing while scanning is in progress and usually consists of the same controls that are on the operator's console. It also facilitates manipulation of the window width and window level, sagittal and coronal reconstruction, scout-view localization, radiation treatment planning, and multi-format camera recording, and displays stored scans and a number of other image analysis capabilities. A combined operator/diagnostic console is shown in Figure 5–16. Two alphanumeric keyboards are clearly seen.

MULTI-IMAGE MULTI-FORMAT CAMERA

This camera is usually an integral component in a CT system. It is a free-standing component that records images photographically onto x-ray film. The inside of the camera consists of a video display (image) with good image quality and an accurate electro-optical system for recording high quality photographic images.

The film size and image formats will be different for different cameras, but some common formats are shown in Figure 5–17.

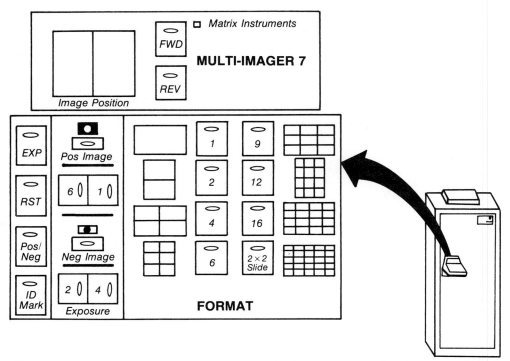

Figure 5–17. Schematic of a multi-image multi-format camera showing a number of different image formats. (Courtesy of Picker International.)

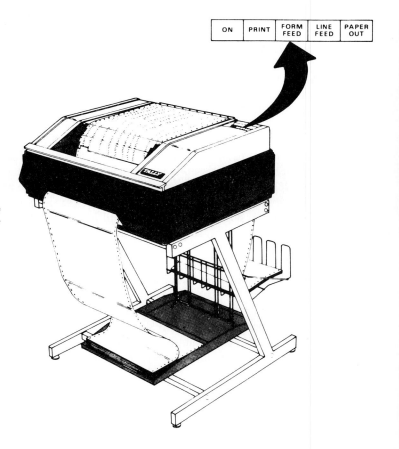

Figure 5–18. A TALLY line printer used in CT. (Courtesy of Picker International.)

THE LINE PRINTER

The line printer was first identified in Chapter 1 (Fig. 1–13) as an output device that prints out a numerical matrix of CT numbers.

The printer shown in Figure 5–18 is used in CT mainly to provide a numerical print-out of the scan (an analysis of the print-out will assist in quantitative assessment of the results of the scan), and to provide a hard-copy listing of the day's work stored on the magnetic tape or disks (e.g., patient names, numbers, date, number of images, etc.).

WINDOW WIDTH AND WINDOW LEVEL

It was pointed out in Chapter 2 that the linear attenuation coefficients of structures within the patient were used by the computer to calculate CT numbers. These numbers are then converted to a gray level scale and displayed on a CRT device for viewing. The gray level can be manipulated to provide optimum demonstration of different structures seen on the image.

In CT, there are two parameters that are extremely important in this regard, since their use is directly controlled by the operator/viewer. These two controls are the window width and window level.

The *window width* (WW) is the range of CT numbers for the gray scale, while the midpoint or center of the gray scale is the *window level* (WL).

By changing the WW and WL, the radiologist can enhance the visualization of structures in which he is most interested. In essence the window width control alters the contrast of the image and the window level the density or CT number of the tissue to be displayed.

In Figure 5–19A, the range of CT numbers (WW) is +1000 (bone) to −1000 (air). The center of that range (WL) is 0 (water). In Figure 5–19B, where the WW is 200 and the WL is 0, all CT numbers more than +100 appear white and those less than −100 appear black, while those between +100 and −100 appear as gray levels. In Figure 5–19C, where the WW is 200 and the WL is +40, the numbers less than −60 appear black, those more than +140 appear white, and those in the range between −60 and +140 appear as gray levels. In Figure 5–19D, where the WW is 400 and the WL is 0, those numbers between +200 and −200 appear as gray levels.

For optimum viewing of an image, the selection of the appropriate WW and WL is usually the choice of the radiologist. This, of course, will depend on the structures examined.

Figure 5–20 shows the effect of different WW and WL settings on several CT scans. The gray scale is displayed on either the right or the left side of the image, with the top and bottom numbers representing the limits of the WW. The WL is also shown on the image. Decreasing the window width enhances the noise.

RESEARCH FINDINGS

Although several measurement modes (areas and mean and standard deviation of CT numbers in any region of interest) exist on some CT machines,

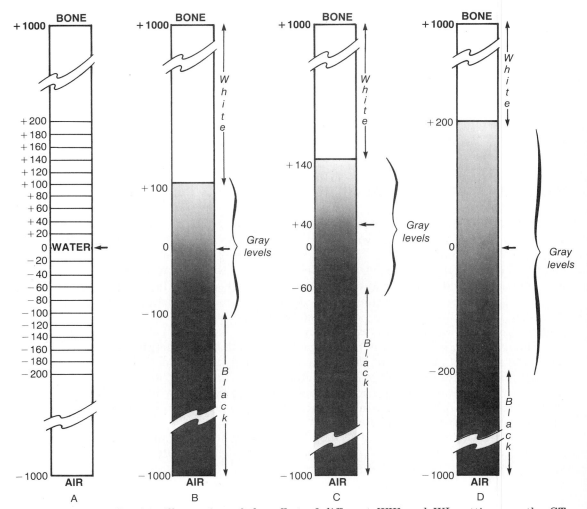

Figure 5-19. Graphic illustration of the effect of different WW and WL settings on the CT image.

an interesting study was done by Koehler et al. (1979) to investigate the effect of window controls on anatomical measurements from the CT scan.

Several special phantoms were made for the study and measurements were made using a number of window settings. The reader should refer to the methodology for more details of the study.

Some of the results of this investigation indicate that:

1. WL position influences the dimensions of anatomical structures. This is illustrated in Figure 5-21.

2. WW changes do not significantly affect these dimensions.

3. "In general, it appears that the larger the density (CT number) difference between two areas involved in the measurement estimate, the greater the potential error. Small lesions are subject to larger percentage errors in measurement than larger ones" (Koehler et al., 1979).

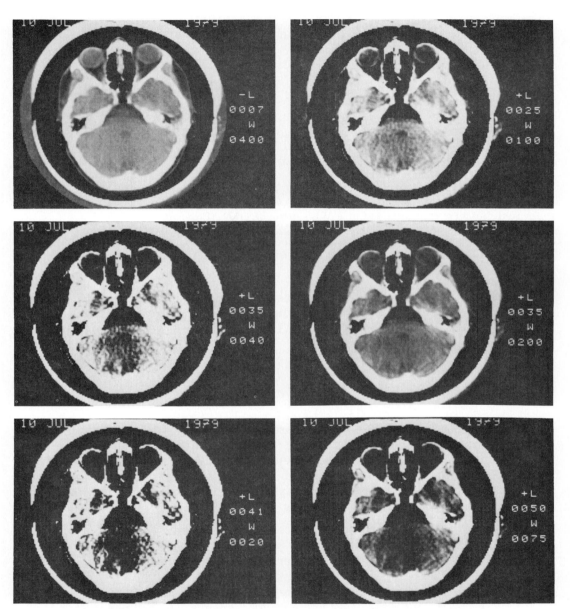

Figure 5–20. The effect of several WW and WL settings on the CT scans.

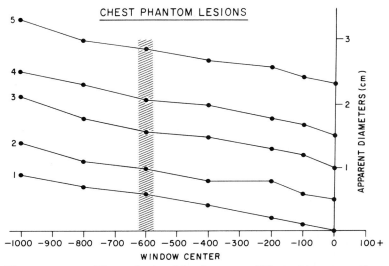

Figure 5-21. The relationship between WL settings on the diameters of chest phantom lesions. The shaded portion represents the actual diameter that occurred at a WL setting of −600. (From Koehler, P. R., Anderson, R. E., and Baxter, B.: The effect of computed tomography viewer controls on anatomical measurements. Radiology, *130*:189, 1979. Reproduced by permission.)

Another study relating to measurement and position of the WL is one by Fullerton et al. (1978). The investigators found that errors can arise in image contour measurement when the WL is set higher or lower than some "optimum value."

THE WATER BOX IN CT

The original EMI scanner used a box in which the patient's head was surrounded by water for the scan (Fig. 5–22). The front of the box is a rubber diaphragm that fits over the patient's head. Prior to scanning, the box is filled with water so that the diaphragm collapses to fit tightly around the head.

The use of this technique ensures a higher degree of accuracy during scanning because of the following:

1. The radiation beam passes through the same thickness of water and object (head), as can be seen in Figure 5–22*B* (Brooks and DiChiro, 1976a).
2. The removal of air between the head and detectors.
3. The reduction of beam-hardening effects.
4. The acquisition of accurate transmission readings.
5. Having water as a reference for transmission readings in each view.
6. Restriction of the dynamic range of the detectors. Such restriction "reduces non-linearity and instability problems" (Phelps et al., 1975).

The water bag has now been eliminated on most CT scanners and has been replaced by wedges, which basically serve the same purpose as the water bag except that the wedges do not totally correct for beam-hardening artifacts. These artifacts can be reduced or eliminated using special computer software.

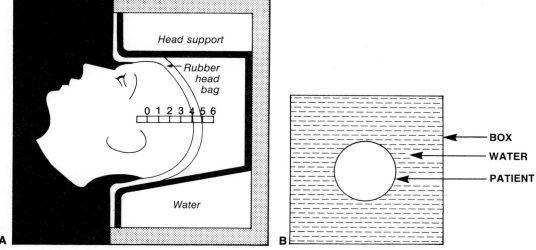

Figure 5–22.   Head of patient positioned in water box (*A*) (Courtesy of EMI Medical, Inc.). Schematic of how the box provides symmetrical geometry (*B*).

Such methods are now being used by some CT equipment manufacturers (Brooks and DiChiro, 1976a).

PERFORMANCE EVALUATION AND QUALITY ASSURANCE

One other important aspect of equipment is that of performance evaluation and quality assurance, as these are receiving more and more attention by radiation control agencies and other related groups. It is also of importance, since equipment efficiency, consistency, and safety coupled with high quality images acquired with the use of minimal radiation doses are of concern to radiologists.

PERFORMANCE EVALUATION

The American Association of Physicists in Medicine (AAPM) identifies performance as a "measurement of a system's capability" (AAPM, 1977).

Several parameters used in evaluation include contrast scale, spatial resolution, precision (noise), linearity, artifacts, and patient exposure. A discussion of all these parameters is not within the scope of this section, and the reader should refer to several interesting works (MacIntyre et al., 1976; McCullough et al., 1974, 1976; Brooks and DiChiro, 1976b) for further information. However, definitions of several of these parameters are given in Table 5–2.

The Bureau of Radiological Health (BRH) of the U.S. Department of Health and Human Services has already prepared drafts on performance standards for CT equipment (FDA-BRH, 1978). The drafts deal with information pertaining to definitions, conditions of operation, dose and imaging performance information, and quality assurance.

TABLE 5–2.   DEFINITIONS OF SEVERAL PARAMETERS USED IN
PERFORMANCE EVALUATION OF CT EQUIPMENT

PARAMETER	DEFINITION
Contrast scale	The change in linear attenuation coefficient per CT number
Spatial resolution	The ability to distinguish two objects from each other in a noiseless field
Noise (precision)	A variation of CT numbers around some average or mean value when scanning a uniform material (e.g., a water bath)
Linearity	An expression to establish whether CT numbers vary in a linear fashion with the linear attenuation coefficients of the material studied

From American Association of Physicists in Medicine: Report No. 1. Phantoms for performance evaluation and quality assurance of CT scanners. Chicago, Ill., American Association of Physicists in Medicine, 1977.

QUALITY ASSURANCE

Quality assurance in CT (as in conventional imaging) refers to tests which indicate that equipment performance is acceptable and consistent.

In the development of performance standards and quality assurance in CT, numerous phantoms have been designed to carry out the appropriate testing. The AAPM Report (1977) on "phantoms for performance evaluation and quality assurance of CT scanners" identifies a number of phantoms and discusses their use in CT. Such phantoms include sections to determine noise, contrast scale, spatial resolution, and linearity. Other phantoms and their use are given by McCullough (1978) and Bellon et al. (1979).

McCullough (1978) demonstrated a number of limitations in CT scanner performance. These relate to the inability of the scanner to correct for beam hardening, to recognize the amount of gantry angulation used, and to center properly, and to the production of artifacts by large amounts of bone. The results of the study by Bellon et al. indicate that the use of phantoms is both practical and inexpensive in evaluation of CT scanner performance.

In the future these phantoms will become commonplace in radiology departments, and the technologist will play a more important role in quality assurance in CT. Already technologists conduct several simple tests on a daily or weekly basis using phantoms provided by CT equipment manufacturers. Once again, these tests are to ensure that the scanner functions accurately and provides consistent results.

Actual tests performed will not be treated here, since each CT system will have its own characteristic test procedure using a number of different parameters. One such test is given in Table 5–3. In Table 5–4, a number of other quality assurance tests is shown. Although these tests were done on an American Science and Engineering CT unit, the authors (Cacak and Hendee, 1979) report that they "should prove useful in establishing quality control programs for other CT scanners." More recently (1981), three more important quality assurance tests (see Appendix B, p. 122) have been added to the list given in Table 5–4.

TABLE 5–3. PHANTOM SCAN CHECK FOR SYNERVIEW CT SYSTEM*

| | SETTINGS | |
PARAMETER	*Half Field*	*Full Field*
1. Field size	24 cm. or smaller	25 cm. or larger
2. Table index	0	0
3. kV	130	130
4. mA	65	95
5. Scan speed	2	2
6. Window width	250	250
7. Window level	0	0

Use the cursor to check that the density is consistently zero in the water areas. A profile may be displayed. It must be flat in the water areas.

*This check is to be done daily on the water phantom. The phantom is positioned on the patient's couch in the x-ray beam plane. (Quoted from SYNERVIEW operator's guide and reproduced by permission of Picker International.)

TABLE 5–4. QUALITY ASSURANCE TESTS FOR CT

TEST	FREQUENCY OF TEST	PHANTOM	PARAMETERS TO BE MEASURED	RATIONALE
1. CT number of water	Daily	8-inch water phantom	CT number in center	Tests for CT number consistency. Departures from zero for water may indicate kVp drift or algorithm misadjustment.
			Standard deviation of CT number	Standard deviation should be constant. Departures from constancy may indicate that tube output is changing, mA drift, or that algorithm is changing. Sharp rises in S.D. may indicate that x-ray tube is near fail point (i.e., output is low).
2. CT number of other materials	Daily	Phantom containing several types of plastic	CT number for each plastic	Test for CT number constancy. Changes in slope may indicate kVp drift or algorithm misadjustment.
3. High-contrast resolution	Daily	High contrast hole phantom or star phantom	Number of sets of holes visible	Test for resolution performance. This test is not very sensitive and resolution must vary substantially before it can be detected. Ideally, an MTF test should be performed daily, but this is impractical without some computer automation.
4. Hard-copy output tests	Daily	Image of phantom or patient stored in memory or gray scale image, if available	Optical density of gray scale in midrange	Tests the overall density of the hard-copy image. Adjust hard-copy device as necessary in case of drift. Most frequently problems are processor related.
			Optical density at each end of gray scale	Tests for contrast constancy. Adjust hard copy in case of drift. Again, beware of processor drifts!
5. Low-contrast resolution	Bi-weekly	Low-contrast phantom $\Delta\mu = 0.5\%$	Number of holes visible	Test for low contrast resolution. This test is similar to Test No. 3 and is not very sensitive. Usually a degradation of low contrast resolution is caused by increase in noise which may be detected by Test No. 1, second parameter.

Table continued on following page

TABLE 5–4. QUALITY ASSURANCE TESTS FOR CT *(Continued)*

TEST	FREQUENCY OF TEST	PHANTOM	PARAMETERS TO BE MEASURED	RATIONALE
6. Image distortion	Bi-weekly	Image distortion phantom	Check image for astigmatism and distortion by physically measuring distance between holes. Measure vertically and horizontally.	The distance between any two adjacent holes (or "dots") on image should be identical. If not, image possesses astigmatism. This test is particularly important if CT images are used for radiation therapy treatment planning.
			Check distance indicators for accuracy	Distance indicators should be acurate at all image magnification.
7. Patient dosimetry	Bi-monthly	TLD phantom, segmented ion chamber or film	Dose profile	Shift in dose profile may be due to a shift in collimation system or change in tube output. Latter may be due to changing tube conditions (aging) or mA changes.
8. Artifact generation	Bi-monthly	Artifact phantom	Qualitatively assess the artifacts and compare with earlier results.	A change in the amount of artifact may indicate mechanical and/or algorithm misalignment.
9. Bed indexing	Bi-monthly	Pre-wrapped film	Accuracy of bed increment	Accuracy should be measured for several increments of most commonly used values of increments.
			Bed reproducibility	Move bed several steps in both directions, ultimately stopping at point at which bed position indicator was started. Check to make sure that bed has actually returned to original position.
10. Misc. CT number checks	Semi-annually	Water phantoms of various sizes	CT number shift with phantom size. Shift with slice width. Shift with reconstruction algorithm type. Shift with position of phantom in scan circle. Shift as position within phantom varies	Establish whether there are CT number shifts as technique is changed. Correct the shifts with hardware and software adjustments if possible. Otherwise establish additive corrections to be made to the absolute value of CT number. Advise users of these corrections.
11. kVp and mA waveforms	Annually or as needed	High-voltage divider and oscilloscope	Measure amplitude and shape of kVp and mA waveforms	Compare results with previous waveform shapes and calibrate HV generator to required kVp and mA accuracy if necessary.

From Cacak, R. K., and Hendee, W. R.: Performance evaluation of a fourth-generation computed tomography (CT) scanner. Proceed. SPIE: Vol. 173, Application of Optical Instrumentation in Medicine VII. Washington, D.C., Society of Photo-Optical Instrumentation Engineers, 1979. Reproduced by permission.

Apart from conducting these simple tests on the equipment, the CT technologist is responsible for a number of other equally important maintenance procedures. These include (a) cleaning the read/write heads and the path through which the tape is threaded with isopropyl alcohol, and (b) cleaning and checking photographic recording equipment. Instructions on these duties are given in equipment manuals.

ROOM FACILITIES FOR CT EQUIPMENT

The installation of CT equipment requires many kinds of personnel in the planning process and careful consideration of room layout.

SITE PLANNING

Site planning calls for a close working relationship among architects, engineers, physicists, purchasers of the equipment, and manufacturers. Careful planning and design of CT facilities ensures the following:

1. Efficient functioning of all components of the CT system.
2. Efficient management of the workload (includes management of the patient).
3. Efficient utilization of the available space.
4. Proper design for shielding against radiation.

The role of each individual in CT site planning is important. For example, the architect examines structural engineering and floor space requirements and other related matters (future plans, methods to reduce the noise level —an acoustical ceiling, for example). In some cases he may also study the general electrical and air-conditioning requirements, or these may be done by the equipment manufacturer.

The purchaser forms a group of people who will eventually influence the acquisition of a CT scanner. Such people (in a hospital) may be the administrator, the radiologist, the radiation physicist, and chief technologist. Administration provides the money for the purchase, while the radiologist and chief technologist play a role in furnishing data concerning the workload, patient flow, etc.

It is the responsibility of the radiation physicist to assist in the proper design of radiation protective shielding and careful arrangement of the equipment, to ensure maximum radiation protection of patients and personnel. These duties having been performed, blueprints and specifications are prepared for approval by the purchaser.

ROOM LAYOUT

The room layout will differ from institution to institution because of different needs and requirements. A typical layout for a CT room calls for a division of the room into three sections to house different components of the equipment. These sections are:

a. The *scanning room,* which generally houses the scanning gantry and patient couch. Such a room should be large enough to allow for easy manipulation of stretchers and emergency equipment.

b. The *computer room,* which houses the CPU and other peripheral equipment.

c. The *control room,* which houses the x-ray control unit, the photographic recording equipment, and the control and viewing consoles. In some instances the computer and control rooms may be combined into one room.

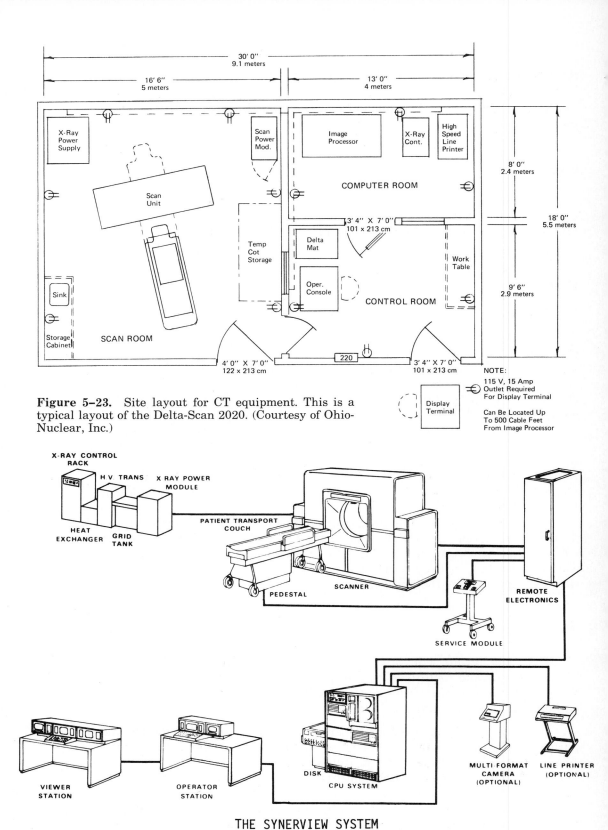

Figure 5–23. Site layout for CT equipment. This is a typical layout of the Delta-Scan 2020. (Courtesy of Ohio-Nuclear, Inc.)

THE SYNERVIEW SYSTEM

Figure 5–24. Relationships of various components in a CT system. (Courtesy of Picker International.)

Figure 5–23 shows a site layout which is divided into the three sections mentioned above. It is also important to note the inclusion of a worktable, a storage cabinet, and a sink in the CT room, as these are very useful to radiologic personnel.

The components discussed in this chapter are all important in the total performance of a CT system. The basic operation of a CT unit involves input, processing, and output. Figure 5–24 illustrates a general scheme of one CT system, showing how each component is related to the total unit.

CT / 5

SUMMARY/REFERENCES/BIBLIOGRAPHY/REVIEW QUESTIONS/APPENDIX

Summary

1. There are three major components in a CT system. These are the imaging component, the computer, and the image display and recording components.

2. The imaging system includes the x-ray tube and detectors, which are mounted in a gantry. Characteristics of the gantry such as aperture and degree of tilt are discussed briefly.

3. The computer system processes information from the detectors to reconstruct the CT image. A number of tasks that are performed by the computer are pointed out. The CPU and input/output devices are identified.

4. Image display is achieved through the control and viewing console.

5. Image documentation in CT can be done either on film or by video recording on magnetic data carriers.

6. Film documentation includes instant-picture photography and wet-processing, while video recording of analog information is done on magnetic tape, disks, or floppy diskettes.

7. An interesting note (the work of Winter, 1978) on television artifacts due to nonsynchronization of camera exposures and the television sweep is mentioned. These artifacts include the appearance of dark and bright bands on the CT photographic image.

8. Some characteristic features of CT control consoles are the control panel, alphanumeric keyboard, CRT display device, photographic recording equipment, floppy disk drive, interactive function keys, and other controls such as the joystick and trackball. A short explanation of each is given.

9. A number of optional CT equipment accessories are commercially available. Only two of these are discussed here. The multi-image multi-format camera uses x-ray film for recording. A number of different film sizes and image formats can be used, depending on the unit. The line printer produces a numerical print-out of the CT image and can also provide a listing of all patients examined, including such data as date, age, sex, and number.

10. The window width is the range of CT numbers in an image, whereas the window level represents the center or midpoint of the range. The window width control essentially changes the image contrast.

11. Some research findings with respect to the effect of window controls on anatomical measurements are presented briefly.

12. Some CT units utilize a water bath. The purpose of such a water bath is discussed.

13. Performance evaluation and quality control in CT are introduced by stating several parameters used in both. Room facilities for CT equipment involve planning and site layout. Planning includes the integration of expertise from the architect, the radiologist, the chief technologist, the radiation physicist, the purchaser of the equipment, and the manufacturer.

14. Careful planning ensures efficient operation, patient management, and radiation safety.

15. Usually, a typical layout for a CT room divides the room into three sections — the scanning room, the computer room, and the control room.

References

American Association of Physicists in Medicine: Report No. 1. Phantoms for Performance Evaluation on Quality Assurance of CT Scanners. Chicago, Ill., American Association of Physicists in Medicine, 1977.

Banna, M.: Basic introduction to computerized tomography. J. Can. Assoc. Radiol., 27:143–147, September, 1976.

Bellon, E. M., Miraldi, F. D., and Wiesen, E. J.: Phantom-model evaluation of CT scanner performance. Applied Radiol., 53–56, July-August, 1979.

Brooks, R. A., and DiChiro, G.: Principles of computer assisted tomography (CAT) in radiographic and radioisotopic imaging. Phys. Med. Biol., 21(5):690–732, 1976a.

Brooks, R. A., and DiChiro, G.: Statistical limitations in x-ray reconstructive tomography. Med. Phys., 21:390–398, 1976b.

Cacak, R. K., and Hendee, W. R.: Performance evaluation of a fourth-generation computed tomography (CT) scanner. Proceed. SPIE: Vol. 173, Application of Optical Instrumentation in Medicine VII. Washington, D.C., Society of Photo-Optical Instrumentation Engineers, 1979.

Cacak, R. K.: Personal communications. University of Colorado Health Sciences Center. Denver, Colorado 30262, December, 1981.

EMI-Medical, Inc.: EMI Scanner 7070 Standard Components — Product Specifications. No. 371. Northbrook, Ill., August 6, 1978.

EMI-Medical, Inc.: Brochure on G. N. Hounsfield's Original Lathe Bed Scanner. Northbrook, Ill., 1979.

Food and Drug Administration — Bureau of Radiological Health (HEW): Proposed Amendment to the Performance Standard for Diagnostic X-ray Equipment Concerning Computed Tomography X-ray Systems. Draft No. 2, October 23, 1978.

Fullerton, G. D., Sewchand, W., Payne, J. T., et al.: CT determination of parameters for inhomogeneity correction in radiation treatment therapy of the esophagus. Radiology, 126:167–171, 1978.

Koehler, P. R., Anderson, R. E., and Baxter, B.: The effect of computed tomography viewer controls on anatomical measurements. Radiology, 130:189–194, 1979.

Krumme, H. J.: A new computerized tomographic head unit: The Siretom 2000. Electromedica, 3–4:123–128, 1977.

MacIntyre, W. J., et al.: Comparative modulation transfer functions of the EMI and Delta scanners. Radiology, 120:189–191, 1976.

McCullough, E. C.: Factors affecting the use of quantitative information from a CT scanner. Radiology, 124:99–107, 1977.

McCullough, E. C.: Anthropomorphic phantoms for computed tomography scanner performance evaluation. J. Comput. Assist. Tomogr., 2:109–112, 1978.

McCullough, E. C., et al.: An evaluation of the quantitative features of a scanning x-ray transverse axial tomograph: The EMI scanner. Radiology, 111:709–715, 1974.

McCullough, E. C., Payne, J. T., et al.: Performance evaluation and quality assurance of computed tomography scanners with illustrations from EMI, Acta and Delta scanners. Radiology, 120:173–188, 1976.

Phelps, M. E., Hoffman, E. J., Gado, M., and Ter-Pogossian, M. M.: Computerized transaxial transmission reconstructive tomography. In DeBlanc, H. J., and Sorenson, J. A. (Eds.): Non-Invasive Brain Imaging. New York, Society of Nuclear Medicine, 1975.

Weckesser, W. D., Scharl, P., and Krumme, H. J.: CT image documentation — state of the art and outlook. Electromedica, 4:122–127, 1978.

Weinstein, M., Berlin, A., Jr., and Duchesneau, P.: High resolution computed tomography of the orbit with the Ohio Nuclear Delta head scanner. Am. J. Roentgenol., 127:175–177, 1976.

Winter, J.: Television display synchronization artifact. Am. J. Roentgenol., 130:373–374, 1978.

Bibliography

Koehler, P. R., Anderson, R. E., and Baxter, B.: The effect of computed tomography viewer controls on anatomical measurements. Radiology, 130:189–194, 1979.

McCullough, E. C.: Factors affecting the use of quantitative information from a CT scanner. Radiology, 124:99–107, 1977.

McCullough, E. C., Payne, J. T., et al.: Performance evaluation and quality assurance of computed tomography scanners with illustrations from EMI, Acta and Delta scanners. Radiology, 120:173–188, 1976.

Weckesser, W. D., Scharl, P., and Krumme, H. J.: CT image documentation — state of the art and outlook. Electromedica, 4:122–127, 1978.

Review Questions

1. Which of the following components compose the imaging system in CT?
   (a) The control and storage devices
   (b) The x-ray tube and detectors
   (c) CRT display devices
   (d) The central processing unit

2. The structure which houses the x-ray tube and detectors in CT is:
   (a) The scanning gantry.
   (b) The x-ray tube housing.
   (c) The detector housing.
   (d) The central processing unit.

3. The contrast of the CT image is essentially controlled by:
   (a) The window width control.
   (b) The joystick.
   (c) The kVp meter.
   (d) The mA setting.

4. If the window width setting is 200 and the window level is 0, which of the following occurs?
   (a) CT numbers greater than +100 appear white.
   (b) CT numbers less than −100 appear gray.
   (c) CT numbers between 0 and +200 appear black.
   (d) Only those numbers between +100 and +200 appear gray.

5. The water bath in CT does not:
   (a) Reduce beam-hardening artifacts.
   (b) Use water as a reference for transmission readings.
   (c) Get rid of air between the patient's head and rubber bag.
   (d) Immobilize the patient's head.

6. Beam-hardening artifacts cannot be reduced or eliminated by using:
   (a) A water bath.
   (b) Pre-processing filter techniques.
   (c) Post-processing correction techniques.
   (d) Appropriate WW and WL settings.

7. A change in the linear attenuation coefficient per CT number relative to water is defined as:
   (a) Linearity.
   (b) The contrast scale.
   (c) Precision.
   (d) Accuracy.

8. Which is used to record the video signal in CT?
   (a) A Polaroid camera
   (b) A Nikon camera
   (c) Magnetic tape
   (d) X-ray film

9. The WW and WL settings for a given CT examination of the abdomen are 400 and 0, respectively. Which of the following is true?
   (a) All structures between +200 and −200 will spread through the gray scale.
   (b) All structures between +200 and −200 will be white.
   (c) All structures between +200 and −200 will be black.
   (d) Only those structures above 400 will have different shades of gray.

10. The concept of real time processing in CT implies:
    (a) That viewing of the image is possible only when scanning is complete.
    (b) That viewing of the image is possible during the scanning sequence.
    (c) That image reconstruction occurs only when the x-ray tube is not energized.
    (d) That images can be recorded very quickly.

11. Which of the following permits the technologist to enter information relating to the patient and scanning process into the computer?
    (a) The CRT device on the operator console
    (b) Floppy disks
    (c) The line printer
    (d) The alphanumeric keyboard on the operator's console

12. Which of the following is *not* true for magnetic storage in CT?
    (a) Retrieval time for acquisition of stored images is long.
    (b) Retrieval time for accessing stored images is short.
    (c) Cost is low.
    (d) It is sensitive to environmental changes.

13. The floppy disk in CT is:
    (a) An example of a secondary storage device.
    (b) An example of a primary storage device.
    (c) Designed to record images off the multi-image multi-format camera.
    (d) An example of an output device in a computer system.

14. Which of the following viewing modes provides important statistical data (mean, standard deviation, etc.) relating to a portion of a CT image?
    (a) ROI
    (b) Highlight
    (c) Scannogram
    (d) Point-to-point

15. The viewing mode which distinguishes tissues of similar densities by making more conspicuous a certain range of CT numbers is the:
    (a) ROI.
    (b) Point-to-point.
    (c) Scout view localization.
    (d) Highlight.

Appendix A

CHARACTERISTICS OF DIFFERENT CT SCANNERS AND THEIR RESPECTIVE MANUFACTURERS

COMPANY	MODEL	APPLICATION	DETECTORS PER SLICE	WATER BAG	ANGULAR MOTION	MATRIX SIZE	PIXEL SIZE (mm)	SCAN TIME	ADDITIONAL PROCESSING TIME‡
I. One detector — two motions									
EMI	Mark I, CT1000	Head	1 NaI†	Yes	180/225° in 1° steps	160	1.5	4.5 min.	30 s
Hitachi	CT-H250	Head	1 NaI†	Yes	180° in 1° steps	256	1	4 min.	0
CGR	Densitome	Head	1 prop.†	No	180° in 1° steps	128	2	4 min.	0
Pfizer	ACTA 0100, 0200	Body	1 CaF₂†	No	180° in 1 or 2° steps	160/320	1.5*	4.5 min.	0
II. Multidetectors — two motions									
General Electric	CT/N(II)	Head	3 NaI†	No	180° in 3° steps	160	1.5	2 min.	30 s
Siemens	Siretom II	Head	4 CaF₂†	No	180° in 1–35° steps	256	1*	1.3 min.	0
Ohio Nuclear	Δ-Scan 25	Head	7 BGO†	No	196° in 7° steps	256	1*	1/3 min.	0
EMI	CT1010	Head	8 NaI†	No	180/225° in 3° steps	320	0.75	1/4.5 min.	90 s
Ohio Nuclear	Δ-Scan 50	Body	3 CaF₂†	No	180° in 3° steps	256	0.75–1.75*	2–2.5 min.	0
Ohio Nuclear	Δ-Scan 50 Fast	Body	12 BGO†	No	180° in 12° steps	256	1/1.7*	18 s	15 s
Syntex	60	Body	12 NaI	Opt.	180° in 12° steps	256	1/1.5*	1 min.	2.5 min.
EMI	CT5000, 5005	Body	30 NaI	No	180° in 10° steps	320	0.75/1/1.25	20 s	3.3 min.
Pfizer	ACTA 0200 FS	Body	30 CaF₂	No	180/280° in 20° steps	160/256/320	1/1.5	21 s	5 s
Philips	Tomoscan	Body	30 BGO	No	180/225° in 10° steps	256	1/1.6/2*	27 s	5 s
Elscint	Scanex	Body	60 BGO	No	180° in 30° steps	256/512	0.5/2*	10 s	10 s
III. Multidetectors — one motion (rotation)									
Artronix	1110	Head	128 Xe	Yes	360° continuous	256	1*	9 s	1.5 min.
General Electric	CT/M	Breast	111 Xe	Yes	360° continuous	128	1.5	10 s	1.7 min.
Picker	Synerview	Body	60 CaF₂	No	720° continuous	240	1/2*	10 s	30 s
Searle	Photrax	Body	252 Xe	No	360° continuous	256	0.5/1/2	5/10/20 s	40 s
Mass. Gen. Hosp.	CTC	Body	256 Xe	No	360° continuous	320	0.8/1.6	5 s	1 min.
Varian		Body	300 Xe–Kr	No	360° continuous	256	1.9*	6 s	2 min.
General Electric	CT/T	Body	320 Xe	No	360° continuous	320	1.3*	5 s	3.3 min.
Artronix	1120	Body	512 Xe	No	360° continuous	512	1*	5 s	3 min.
Am. Sci. & Eng.		Body	600 BGO	No	495° continuous	512	0.5/1*	5/10/20 s	1 min.

*Magnification mode available to display sub-portion of image on full matrix.
†Scans two slices simultaneously; thus total number of signal detectors is double.
‡Before first image can be displayed.
From Brooks, R. A., and DiChiro, G.: Principles of computer assisted tomography (CAT) in radiographic and radioisotopic imaging. Phys. Med. Biol., 21(5):690–732, 1976. Reproduced by permission.

Appendix B

OTHER QUALITY ASSURANCE TESTS IN CT*

TEST	FREQUENCY OF TEST	PHANTOM	PARAMETERS TO BE MEASURED	RATIONALE
Light field indicator alignment	Bi-monthly	Pre-wrapped film with pin holes	Location of scan slice relative to light indicator	Center of radiation within 2 mm of light indicator.
Collimator checks	Annually or as performance evaluation	Beam width phantom	Beam width or "sensitivity profile" at several collimator settings	Check if the sensitivity profile matches the dose profile. Dose profile may be significantly larger on some CT units. Sensitivity profile FWHM should closely approximate the nominal collimator setting over range of adjustments.
Noise/ dose characteristics	Annually or as performance evaluation	8-inch water phantom	Measure noise (standard deviation, σ) as a function of dose, D, and beam width, w.	Standard Deviation should approximate the relation: $$\sigma = \text{constant}/\sqrt{D_w}$$

*These tests were provided through the courtesy of R. K. Cacak, Ph.D., of the University of Colorado Health Sciences Center, Denver, Colorado, and reproduced by permission.

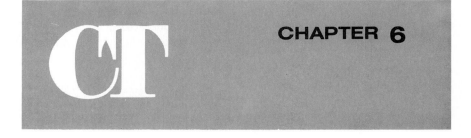

CHAPTER 6

IMAGE QUALITY

The quality of the CT image can be completely described in terms of spatial resolution and contrast resolution.

DOUGLAS P. BOYD (1977)

When an x-ray beam enters an object, it is attenuated by its passage through the object. The beam that emerges contains information about the structures in that object. Such information (a distribution of radiation intensities), when received by a suitable detector (e.g., film), generates an *x-ray image*.

In CT, this information is received by either an ionization or a scintillation detector, which converts the x-ray image into electrical signals that are fed into the computer for processing.

QUALITIES OF THE IMAGE

DEFINITION OF QUALITY

Image quality in CT refers to how clearly and faithfully structures in the image can be visualized. As indicated previously, this image is displayed on a TV monitor and is available for film recording. The quality of this display and the final film recording are also important for overall image quality.

123

FACTORS AFFECTING QUALITY

In conventional x-ray imaging, there are a number of factors influencing image quality. Such factors relate to processing, geometry, motion, subject contrast, film contrast, technique, image receptor, focal spot size, viewing conditions, and observer performance.

In CT, there are also several factors affecting image quality (Fig. 6–1). These include (a) measuring errors, (b) representational errors, (c) positioning errors, and (d) image discontinuity errors (Pfieler et al., 1976). For the sake of simplicity, only three factors will be discussed here, as these have been described recently in the scientific literature.

The general expression for image quality as pointed out by Stapleton (1976) is

$$\text{Image quality } \alpha \; \frac{\text{sharpness}^2 \times \text{contrast}^2}{\text{noise power}}$$

Each of these will now be discussed in this chapter.

MEASUREMENT OF IMAGE QUALITY

Several methods can be used to describe certain parameters of image quality. Methods of quantifying resolution include the point spread function (PSF), the line spread function (LSF), the contrast transfer function (CTF), and the modulation transfer function (MTF).

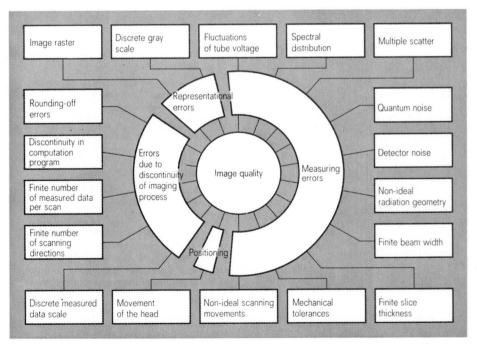

Figure 6–1. Factors affecting the quality of the image in CT. (From Pfeiler, M., Schwierz, G., and Linke, G.: Some guiding ideas on image recording in computerized axial tomography. Electromedica, *1*:19–25, 1976. Reproduced by permission.)

The PSF describes the unsharpness that results when a point in the object is not reproduced as a "true" point in the image. This unsharpness results in a blurring effect (i.e., a spreading-out of the point image to form a measurable circle).

The LSF also describes the unsharpness of an imaging system, when a line or slit object is not reproduced as a line or slit image but rather is spread out over a measureable distance.

The CTF, also referred to as the contrast response function (CRF), is used to measure the contrast response of an imaging system. For the image of a resolution test pattern (series of slits and spaces), the resultant contrast is the difference in density between adjacent regions of the slits. If a graph is plotted between the resultant contrast of the image slits as a function of the number of slits per unit length, the CTF will be obtained. Image contrast decreases as the number of slits per unit length decreases.

The MTF can be derived from the LSF or PSF through Fourier transformation. The MTF is used to measure the resolution capabilities of a system by breaking down an object into its *frequency components*. The MTF at different frequencies can be 1, 0, or some value between 0 and 1. An MTF of 1 implies that the imaging system has exactly reproduced the object, whereas an MTF of 0 indicates no transfer of object to image. A further understanding of the MTF will require a discussion of the physics and mathematics of the curve, which is not within the scope of this chapter.

MTF is important, since it is being used in performance evaluation of CT scanners. Figure 6–2 gives an illustration of the PSF, LSF, and MTF.

Finally, the noise element in an image can be measured by the *noise power spectrum* (Wiener spectrum). This description can be used to study the total noise of the system. Figure 6–3 shows how this spectrum can be obtained, starting from an analysis of the density.

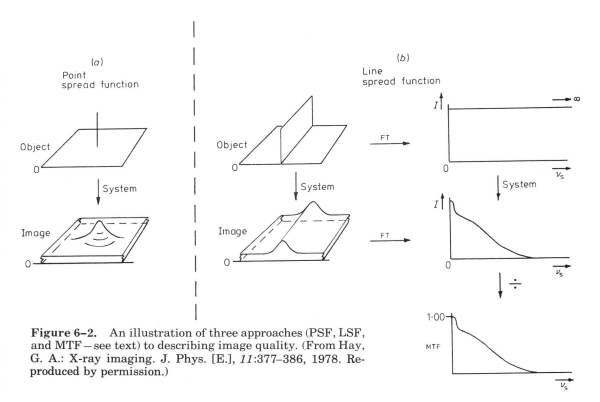

Figure 6–2. An illustration of three approaches (PSF, LSF, and MTF — see text) to describing image quality. (From Hay, G. A.: X-ray imaging. J. Phys. [E.], *11*:377–386, 1978. Reproduced by permission.)

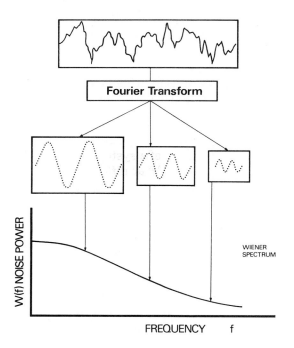

Figure 6–3. A method of obtaining the Wiener spectrum (noise power spectrum). (From Stapleton, R. E.: Image quality in x-ray systems. X-Ray Focus, *14*:46–55, 1976. Reproduced by permission.)

RESOLUTION

Resolution in CT can be discussed in terms of spatial resolution and contrast resolution. Since a description of both topics can become very rigorous, only the more important details will be treated here.

SPATIAL RESOLUTION

Spatial resolution is used to describe the degree of blurring present in an image. It is often represented by the MTF, PSF, or LSF. Several factors that influence spatial resolution are the pixel size, aperture function, data sampling frequency, reconstruction algorithm, and scanning mechanism precision.

The pixel size determines the *display resolution*. The clarity of the image is determined by the number of points in the matrix (Hounsfield, 1978). A matrix of 320×320 (102,400 pixels) improves picture quality over a matrix of 80×80 or 160×160. However, there are a few points to consider:

1. Increasing the number of pixels does not increase the original information or improve the reconstruction resolution (Fig. 6–4*A*).

2. Larger points in the object are enhanced in the image by increasing the number of pixels (Fig. 6–4*B*).

3. Smaller points in the object are not reproduced faithfully and the image on the television monitor screen can be misinterpreted (Fig. 6–4*C*) (Pfeiler et al., 1976).

The *aperture size* refers to the width of the aperture at the detector.

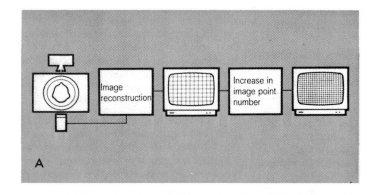

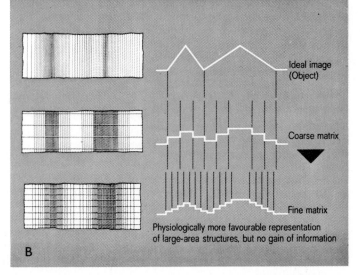

Figure 6–4. Effects of increasing matrix points on resolution. (From Pfeiler, M., Schwierz, G., and Linke, G.: Some guiding ideas on image recording in computerized axial tomography. Electromedica, *1*:19–25, 1976. Reproduced by permission.)

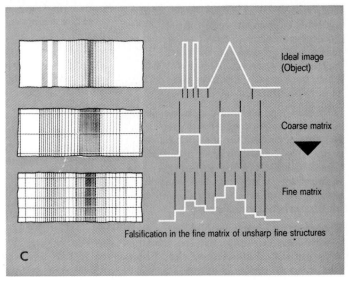

Generally, when the aperture size is smaller than the spacing between objects, the objects can be resolved. This means that for smaller aperture sizes, higher spatial resolution can be obtained.

This effect can be described by the *aperture transfer function* (ATF). A more rigorous treatment of ATF can be found in a paper by Yester and Barnes (1977).

Data sampling frequency relates to the number of transmission readings and the spacing between rays (distance between rays). Greater sampling improves spatial resolution and the overall accuracy of reconstruction.

CONTRAST RESOLUTION

The contrast resolution of a CT scanner is its ability to demonstrate small changes in tissue contrast. This is sometimes referred to as the sensitivity of the CT unit (Hounsfield, 1976).

The density sensitivity of typical CT machines extends from about 0.3 per cent for areas of 1 sq. cm. to 2 per cent for areas of 1 sq. mm. (Boyd, 1977). Most CT scanners should be able to detect tissue differences of about 0.5 per cent in head-sized objects.

Several factors that will affect contrast resolution are the slice thickness, number of photons detected, the size of the television screen (viewer size), and the viewing distance. McCullough (1977) has pointed out that as the viewing distance increases for large TV screens, the ability to detect images of low contrast improves.

Decreasing slice thickness without increasing radiation dose will result in poor quality. On the other hand, increasing photon flux (dose) improves contrast resolution. High contrast resolution CT scans are shown in Figures 6–5 and 6–6.

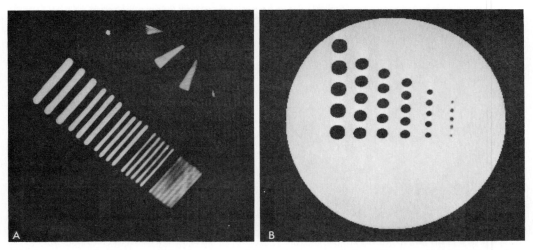

Figure 6–5.   *A*, CT scan of high-contrast line pair gauge of the Alderson CAT-PHAN slices of plastic differing by 500 CT numbers and grouped from 2 to 7 line pairs/cm. Note the visualization of the 7 line pair set, indicating spatial resolution cut-off of greater than 7 line pair/cm. *B*, CT scan of high-contrast resolution insert of the AAPM phantom. Diameters of the air-filled holes are 2.5, 2.0, 1.75, 1.5, 1.25, 1.0, and 0.75 mm., respectively. Note the clear visualization of the 1.0-mm. holes. (These images were obtained on the EMI Scanner 6000. Courtesy of EMI Medical, Inc.)

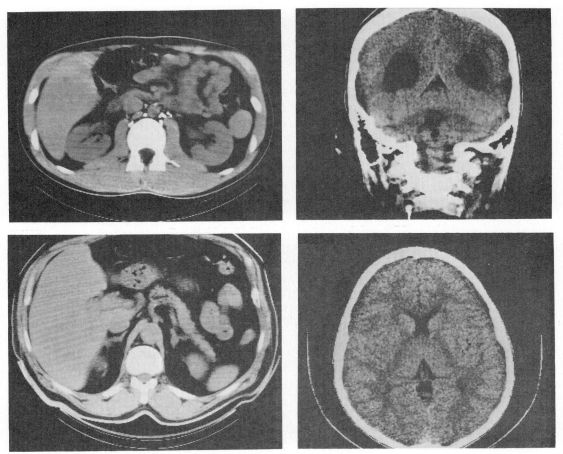

Figure 6–6. High-contrast resolution CT scans. These scans were produced by the General Electric CT/T 8800. (Courtesy of General Electric Medical Systems Division.)

MEASUREMENT OF SPATIAL AND CONTRAST RESOLUTION IN CT

A number of phantoms have been designed to measure spatial and contrast resolution in CT. These phantoms have been used in evaluating CT performance parameters in a number of studies, including those of Judy (1976), MacIntyre et al. (1976), Bischof and Ehrhardt (1977), and Bellon et al. (1979).

Some typical phantoms are:

(a) Contrast scale phantom.

(b) Edge phantom for spatial resolution. This can be used to obtain both the LSF and the MTF as shown by Judy (1977).

(c) Hole phantom for spatial resolution, which consists of a series of carefully arranged holes (of specific sizes) in plexiglass in which water can be placed.

Figure 6–6 shows images of two CT phantoms used for evaluation purposes.

RESEARCH FINDINGS

Bischof and Ehrhardt (1977) investigated the MTF for an EMI CT head scanner with a 160 × 160 matrix. The scanner was operated at 120 kVp and 33 mA with a slice thickness of 1.3 cm. Using a phantom immersed in the water bath, the investigators found the resolution of the scanner to be 3.1 line pairs cm^{-1}.

MacIntyre et al. (1976) and Judy (1976) have also investigated MTF for CT scanners (EMI and Delta Scan). Their results are in close agreement with those of Bischof and Ehrhardt (1977).

The results of Maue-Dickson et al. (1979) indicate that a resolution of 3.7 line pairs was achieved in one system (GE/T 7800), while 6.1 line pairs cm^{-1}. were obtained for another system (GE/T 8800). Another study of interest that should be mentioned here, since it relates to image quality, is one by Prasad (1979), who found that the intensity distribution of the focal spot and the width of the collimator influence resolution in the CT image.

EFFECTS OF MOTION ON IMAGE QUALITY

As in conventional radiography, motion during CT can degrade CT image quality (both spatial and contrast resolution). An interesting study to demonstrate this is one by Alfidi et al. (1976). The workers found that a "variety of periodic and aperiodic physiologic motions" degrades image quality. They found that to improve spatial and contrast resolution, shorter scan times of 2 seconds or less "would appear to be desirable to eliminate" the effects of motion in CT (Alfidi et al., 1976).

NOISE PROPERTIES IN CT

The term *noise* has been mentioned briefly in Chapter 5. In review, the noise in CT is the fluctuation of CT numbers from point to point in the image for a scan of uniform material (e.g., water).

Several papers have been written on noise in CT in which some investigators focused on statistical noise (Chesler et al., 1977; Brooks and DiChiro, 1976) and the noise power spectrum (Riederer et al., 1978).

CT noise can be described using the *standard deviation* (SD) of the values in the image matrix (pixels) using the following expression (Ohio-Nuclear, Inc., 1978):

$$SD = \sqrt{\frac{\sum\limits_{i=1}^{N} (X_i - \overline{X})^2}{N-1}}$$

where N = total number of pixels within the region
$\overline{X}$ = mean of pixels
X_i = individual pixel value

The answer computed will indicate the statistical spread in the reconstructed CT numbers (SD).

The *noise level* can be stated as a percentage of contrast or in CT numbers. In the region of interest (ROI) mode of viewing (Chapter 5), the mean and standard deviation are generally given on one side of the image. If the SD for a system with a CT number range of ± 1000 (Hounsfield scale) is given to be 3, then the noise level expressed as a percentage of contrast is:

$$\text{Noise level } (\%) = \frac{3}{1000} \times 100$$

$$= \frac{3}{10}$$

$$= 0.3\%$$

That is, 3 units out of 1000 represent 0.3% (Ohio-Nuclear, Inc., 1978).

CT scanners will have different noise levels for different modes of operation, object size, matrix size, and radiation dose.

SOURCES OF NOISE

CT noise is mainly related to the following:

1. Number of detected photons
2. Matrix size (pixel size)
3. Slice thickness
4. Algorithm
5. Electronic noise (detector electronics)
6. Scattered radiation
7. Object size

Brooks and DiChiro (1976) have described an expression for noise in CT that shows the relationship of noise to several of the above factors. This mathematical expression is as follows:

$$\sigma\,(\mu)\ \alpha\ \left[\frac{B}{W^3hD_0}\right]^{1/2}$$

where σ = standard deviation
μ = linear attenuation coefficient
B = fractional attenuation through object
W = width of pixel
h = slice thickness
D_0 = entrance dose

A more general relationship of noise to spatial resolution and dose is as follows (Riederer et al., 1978):

$$\sigma^2 \alpha\ 1/N \cdot r^3$$

where σ = standard deviation
N = number of detected primary photons (dose)
r = spatial resolution

The expression indicates that in order to improve spatial resolution by a factor of 2 while keeping σ constant, the dose must be increased by a factor of 8.

One final word on noise which deserves mention here is the *noise power spectrum*. Riederer et al. (1978) point out that:

> Knowledge of the noise power spectrum can be of value 'in understanding the behavior of statistical noise in CT images. The noise power spectrum quantifies the amount of noise at each spatial frequency. Integrating the power spectrum over all frequencies gives an estimate of the variance at any one reconstructed point. Knowledge of the power spectrum enables one to estimate the uncertainty in averages made over regions in CT reconstructions, something which may be important when dealing quantitatively with the reconstructed CT values.

The main point of the power spectrum investigation is that the statistical noise in CT is correlated from point to point (Riederer, 1979).

ARTIFACTS

The appearance of artifacts on a CT image is disturbing and can cause problems in diagnosis. Therefore it is essential that one be able to identify these artifacts, determine their causes, and take the steps necessary to eliminate or reduce them.

The causes of artifacts on the CT image may be related either to the equipment or to the patient.

PATIENT-RELATED ARTIFACTS

The most common of these artifacts are those caused by motion, both voluntary and involuntary. These motion artifacts have been investigated by Alfidi et al. (1976). Any movement during scanning will produce star-like *streaks* on the CT image. These streaks (Fig. 6–7) may appear tangential to the skull or diagonally across the skull for nodding and rotating movements, respectively (Paxton and Ambrose, 1974).

Metallic material on or in the patient generally will produce streak artifacts (Fig. 6–8).

Motion artifacts may be reduced in the following ways:

1. Reduction in scan time below that required to hold a breath.

2. The use of immobilization devices for the head. Such devices are commercially available today.

3. Taking more readings (e.g., rotation of tube and detectors greater than approximately 180° tends to "smooth out" the image).

4. Sedation. Children and patients who are uncooperative or who have been severely traumatized may be sedated; in some cases general anesthesia may be necessary. The type and amount of sedation is left to the physician's discretion.

5. Removal of external metal (necklaces, hairpins, etc.) from the patient.

6. Administration of antiperistaltic drugs.

7. Clear instructions to the patient, stressing the importance of remaining immobile during scanning.

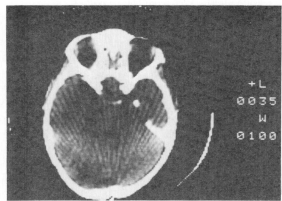

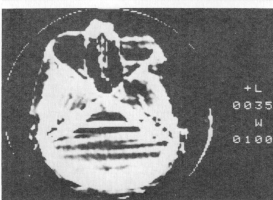

Figure 6–7. Streak artifacts due to patient motion.

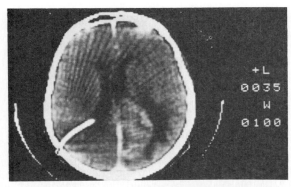

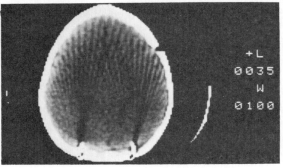

Figure 6–8. Streak artifacts due to the presence of metal in the patient's head.

EQUIPMENT-RELATED ARTIFACTS

Equipment-related artifacts are inevitable, since the system is not perfect (no system is). They are caused by unstable mechanics, detector drift (different detector responses), geometry of the system, changes in photon flux from time to time, insufficient transmission readings, and beam hardening.

The appearance of *ring artifacts* on the CT image may be caused by poorly balanced detectors, detector drift, or spectral changes from time to time. On the other hand, *streak artifacts* may appear; these are related to insufficient sampling (fine streak) and beam hardening (broad streak) (General Electric, 1979).

Another kind of artifact was demonstrated in a study by Goodenough et al. (1975). Their findings indicate that, depending on the slice geometry of the CT system, certain regions of the head will not be imaged during a scan and that there may be overlapping between adjacent slices.

Other artifacts may be caused by particles or water bubbles in the water bath of an EMI Mark I, and air between the water bag and the patient's head ("peacock" artifact) (Huckman et al., 1977).

It is important to realize that many studies and procedures are focused on eliminating or reducing artifacts of the CT image. Such reduction can be obtained by special software corrections and the use of special filter techniques in reconstruction algorithms.

CONTRAST ENHANCEMENT

The term *contrast enhancement* as used in CT refers to a method of improving visualization of certain structures in the CT image through the use of iodinated contrast media.

The early use of contrast in CT began with investigations by Ambrose (1973) and was followed by a number of other studies (e.g., Norton et al., 1978; Messina, 1976; Wing et al., 1976; Davis et al., 1977; York and Marshall, 1975; Kramer et al., 1975; Latchaw et al., 1978; Butler and Kricheff, 1978).

The dose and method of contrast administration are usually based on the physician's judgment, since he is familiar with the patient's clinical history. Two types of dose administration have been investigated. These are:

1. *Bolus injection* (rapid injection), for maximum concentration of the contrast. It has been reported that rapid injection of contrast leads to better vascular visualization.

2. *Infusion method,* in which a large amount of suitable contrast is administered over a period of time. This method is beneficial in evaluation of structural details of lesions.

Contrast enhancement of the CT image is possible with the use of iodinated compounds, since the atomic number for iodine is greater than for soft tissues and bone and since there is increased capillary permeability to iodine (in tumors).

With the administration of contrast media, reactions (allergic or toxic) may occur in the patient. These reactions may result in motion artifacts and may cause discomfort to the patient. Therefore, it is of utmost importance that emergency (life-support) equipment be close at hand.

CT / 6

SUMMARY/REFERENCES/BIBLIOGRAPHY/REVIEW QUESTIONS

Summary

1. The chapter begins with a definition of the x-ray image.
2. The quality of an image is the clarity with which important structures can be visualized.

3. Image quality in CT depends on a number of factors that arise from measurement errors, representational errors, positioning errors, and image discontinuity errors. These are represented in a diagram given by Pfeiler et al. (1976).

4. Several approaches used to describe image quality were discussed briefly as a means of review. These approaches include the line spread function, the point spread function, the contrast transfer function, and the modulation transfer function.

5. Resolution was discussed in terms of spatial resolution and contrast resolution.

6. Spatial resolution is used to describe the degree of unsharpness present in an image. It is often represented by the MTF. Several factors that affect spatial resolution are given.

7. Contrast resolution is the ability of the scanner to detect small changes in tissue density. Several factors that affect contrast resolution in CT include slice thickness, pixel size, detector aperture, and radiation dose.

8. Several phantoms have been designed to measure performance of the CT scanners. These include the contrast scale phantom, the edge phantom for spatial resolution, and the hole phantom for spatial resolution.

9. Some research findings on the MTF for some scanners are presented.

10. The effect of motion on CT images has been found to be degrading. Such effects can be minimized by the use of shorter scan times.

11. Noise in CT can be described by the noise power spectrum. Generally, noise is described by the standard deviation of CT numbers from a scan of water.

12. CT artifacts can be equipment-related or patient-related. Patient motion can produce streak artifacts, while the equipment can produce ring artifacts.

13. Contrast-enhancement in CT refers to the use of contrast media to improve visualization of structures within the patient. Two methods of contrast administration are identified.

References

Alfidi, R. J., MacIntyre, W. J., and Haaga, J. R.: The effects of biological motion on CT resolution. Am. J. Roentgenol., *127*:11–15, 1976.
Ambrose, J.: Computerized transverse axial scanning (tomography). Part 2. Clinical applications. Br. J. Radiol., *46*:1023–1047, 1973.
Bellon, E. M., Miraldi, F. D., and Wiensen, E. J.: Performance evaluation of computed tomography scanners using a phantom model. Am. J. Roentgenol., *132*:345–352, 1979.

Bischof, C. J., and Ehrhardt, J. C.: Modulation transfer function of the EMI CT head scanner. Med. Phys., *4*(2):163–167, 1977.

Boyd, D. P.: Physics II. *In* Norman, D., Korobkin, M., and Newton, T. H. (Eds.): Computed Tomography 1977. St. Louis, The C. V. Mosby Co., 1977.

Brooks, R. A., and Di Chiro, G.: Statistical limitations in x-ray reconstructive tomography. Med. Phys., *21*:390–398, 1976.

Butler, A. R., and Kricheff, I. I.: Non-contrast CT scanning — limited value in suspected brain tumor. Radiology, *126*:689–693, 1978.

Chesler, D. A., Riederer, S. J., and Pelc, N. J.: Noise due to photon counting statistics in computed x-ray tomography. J. Comput. Assist. Tomogr., *1*:64–74, 1977.

Davis, K. R., et al.: Computed tomography of cerebral infarction, hemorrhage, contrast enhancement and time of appearance. Comput. Tomogr., *1*:71–86, 1977.

General Electric: CT/T technology continuum technical performance of the CT/T system. Brochure 4870. General Electric Medical Systems Division, Milwaukee, Wis., 1979.

Goodenough, D. J., Weaver, M. S., and Davis, D. O.: Potential artifacts associated with the scanning pattern of the EMI scanner. Radiology, *117*:615–620, 1975.

Hay, G. A.: X-ray imaging. J. Phys. [E.], *4*:377–386, 1978.

Hounsfield, G. N.: Picture quality of computed tomography. Am. J. Roentgenol., *127*:3–9, 1976.

Hounsfield, G. N.: Potential uses of more accurate CT absorption values by filtering. Am. J. Roentgenol., *131*:103–106, 1978.

Huckman, M. S., Granier, L. S., and Classen, R. C.: The normal computed tomogram. *In* Felson, B.: Computerized Cranial Tomography. New York, Grune and Stratton, 1977.

Judy, P. F.: The line spread function and the modulation transfer function of a computed tomographic scanner. Med. Phys., *3*:233–236, 1976.

Kramer, R. A., et al.: An approach to contrast enhancement in computed tomography of the brain. Radiology, *116*:641–647, 1975.

Latchaw, R. E., et al.: A protocol for the use of contrast enhancement in cranial computed tomography. Radiology, *126*:681–687, 1978.

MacIntyre, W. J., Alfidi, R. J., Haaga, J., Chernak, E., and Meaney, T. F.: Comparative modulation transfer functions of the EMI and Delta scanners. Radiology, *120*:189–191, 1976.

Maue-Dickson, W., Trefler, M., and Dickson, D. R.: Comparison of dosimetry and image quality in computed and conventional tomography. Radiology, *131*:509–514, 1979.

McCullough, E. C.: Factors affecting the use of quantitative information from a CT scanner. Radiology, *124*:99–107, 1977.

Messina, A. V.: Computed tomography-contrast enhancement in intracerebral hemorrhage (abstr.). Neuroradiology, *12*:50, 1976.

Norton, G. A., Kishore P. R. S., and Lin, J.: CT contrast enhancement in cerebral infarction. Am. J. Roentgenol., *131*:881–885, 1978.

Ohio-Nuclear, Inc.: Technical supplement. The Delta Scan 2000 Series of computed tomography scanners. 1978.

Paxton, R., and Ambrose, J.: The EMI scanner. A brief review of the first 650 patients. Br. J. Radiol., *47*:530–565, 1974.

Pfeiler, M., Schwierz, G., and Linke, C. T.: Some guiding ideas on image recording in computerized axial tomography. Electromedica, *1*:19–25, 1976.

Prasad, S. C.: Effects of focal spot intensity distribution and collimation width in reconstructive x-ray tomography. Med. Phys., *6*(3):229–232, 1979.

Riederer, S. J.: Personal communication, 1979.

Riederer, S. J., Pelc, N. J., and Chesler, D. A.: The noise power spectrum in computer x-ray tomography. Phys. Med. Biol., *23*:446–454, 1978.

Stapleton, R. E.: Image quality in x-ray systems. X-ray Focus, *14*:46–55, 1976.

Wing, S. D., et al.: Contrast enhancement of cerebral infarcts — computed tomography. Radiology, *121*:89–92, 1976.

Yester, M. V., and Barnes, G. T.: Geometrical limitations of CT scanner resolution. Proceedings of SPIE/SPSE. Conference on Applications of Optical Instrumentation in Medicine IV. Paper 127–49, September, 1977.

York, D. H., Jr., and Marshall, W. H., Jr.: Recent ischemic brain artifacts in computed tomography: Appearances pre and post-contrast infusion. Radiology, *117*:599–608, 1975.

Bibliography

Alfidi, R. J., MacIntyre, W. J., and Haaga, J. R.: The effects of biological motion on CT resolution. Am. J. Roentgenol., *127*:11–15, 1976.

Boyd, D. P.: Physics II. *In* Norman, D., Korobkin, M., and Newton, T. H., (Eds.): Computed Tomography 1977. St. Louis, The C. V. Mosby Co., 1977.

Goodenough, D. J., Weaver, M. S., and Davis, D. O.: Potential artifacts associated with the scanning pattern of the EMI scanner. Radiology, *117*:615–620, 1975.

Hounsfield, G. N.: Picture quality of computed tomography. Am. J. Roentgenol., *127*:3–9, 1976.

Kramer, R. A., et al.: An approach to contrast enhancement in computed tomography of the brain. Radiology, *116*:641–647, 1975.

McCullough, E. C.: Factors affecting the use of quantitative information from a CT scanner. Radiology, *124*:99–107, 1977.

Pfeiler, M., Schwierz, G., and Linke, G.: Some guiding ideas on image recording in computerized axial tomography. Electromedica, *1*:19–25, 1976.

Review Questions

1. Which of the following will affect image quality in CT?
   (a) Movement of the patient's head
   (b) Slice thickness
   (c) Detector noise
   (d) All of the above

2. Which of the following relates to describing the resolution in an image?
   (a) The PSF
   (b) The LSF
   (c) The MTF
   (d) All of the above

3. Spatial resolution in CT is not related to which of the following?
   (a) The viewing distance
   (b) Pixel size
   (c) Aperture width
   (d) Reconstruction algorithm

4. As given by Hounsfield, which of the following is a measure of picture contrast?
   (a) Sensitivity
   (b) Aperture size
   (c) Slice thickness
   (d) All of the above

5. Which can be used to measure or describe the noise in CT?
   (a) The PSF
   (b) The standard deviation
   (c) The modulation transfer function
   (d) Contrast linearity

6. What is the noise level (%) in a CT unit that uses a number range of ±1000, given that the standard deviation is 5 units?
   (a) 5%
   (b) 0.05%
   (c) 0.5%
   (d) 50%

7. Nodding movements of the patient's head during the CT scanning process result in:
   (a) Streaks tangent to the skull.
   (b) Ring artifacts.
   (c) Diagonal streaks.
   (d) All of the above.

8. Which of the following is not used to reduce motion artifacts caused by the patient?
    (a) Immobilization
    (b) Sedation
    (c) Reduction in scan time
    (d) The use of special filter techniques

9. Contrast enhancement in CT refers to:
    (a) Increasing mA and decreasing kVp.
    (b) The use of contrast media to improve visualization.
    (c) Using special color dyes to enhance the image.
    (d) All of the above.

CT RADIATION DOSE MEASUREMENT
MEASURED CT RADIATION DOSE
CT SCANNER DESIGN PARAMETERS
AFFECTING RADIATION DOSE

CT DOSE IN COMPARISON TO OTHER
DIAGNOSTIC RADIOLOGY DOSES
   Research Findings
   Dose-Reduction Methods

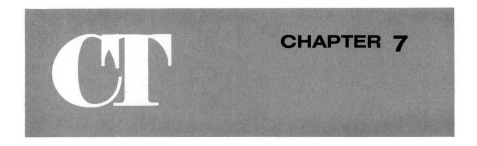

CHAPTER 7

RADIATION DOSE

The maximum surface dosage in most clinical CT scans ranges from 2-10 rads/study but much larger dose per study values seem possible with both rotate-translate and rotary geometry designs. The CT scanner type in itself does not significantly reduce dose.

EDWIN C. McCULLOUGH and J. THOMAS PAYNE (1978)

Computerized tomographic scanning provides the radiologist with true tomographic images of excellent contrast. To obtain this low contrast, a sufficient number of x-ray photons must pass through the region of interest. In spite of statements to the contrary, the patient radiation exposure for a CT scan series usually exceeds that of film radiography of the same area. For various reasons to be discussed, there may be significant differences in patient dosage for different CT scanners. Even though any CT scanner is ultimately governed by the laws of physics, there are over a dozen variables of a CT scan that will affect the patient radiation dose. Variations in collimation, filtration, and x-ray output parameters will result in different radiation doses for different modes of operation. In general, the radiation dose is related primarily to the basic imaging parameters of the CT unit, which include resolution, slice thickness, and noise, and to a lesser extent to collimation, filtration, detector efficiency, and the reconstruction algorithm.

This chapter will provide (1) a description of the methodology for standardized CT dose measurement, (2) CT dose measurements from different CT units, (3) CT scanner design as it relates to radiation dose, and (4) a comparison of CT doses to radiation doses currently employed in the everyday practice of radiology.

CT RADIATION DOSE MEASUREMENT

For a CT scanner, the patient is irradiated with a polychromatic x-ray beam with a distribution of energy from about 20 to 140 kev. The beam quality of the incident beam is in the range of 4 to 8 mm. Al(HVL). Each point of the patient scan surface is also irradiated by emergent x-rays that pass through various lengths of absorber with a higher beam quality. Thus, a radiation dosimeter for CT dose measurements should have a minimum variation in energy sensitivity over a range in beam quality of 4 mm. Al to 1 mm. Cu(HVL).

Furthermore, the CT x-ray beam is highly collimated and generally quite narrow (i.e., 1.5 mm. to 13 mm. for different slice thicknesses). The fact that it is narrow presents a problem of fully irradiating the dosimeter and getting a true response. If one were to use an ionization chamber to measure CT exposure for a 1.5 mm. CT beam, the active volume would have to be very small and therefore have low sensitivity. There is also the practical problem of always placing a small chamber exactly in the center of the small CT beam during the measurement. Recently, Jucius et al. have constructed special long, thin ionization chambers specifically for CT scan exposure measurement. In this case the product of the measured ionization and the active length gives a number related to the exposure at the point of measurement. However, the use of standard ion chambers is precluded. Other dosimeters not restricted by size requirements would include film or thermoluminescent dosimeters (TLD's).

Film is highly energy-sensitive at diagnostic x-ray energies, with an overresponse of as much as 40 times. Thus for the energy range encountered with CT scanners, it would be difficult if not impossible to accurately calibrate film for CT dose measurement. Fortunately, TLD's have a relatively low energy sensitivity over the range encountered in CT scanning. For lithium fluoride (TLD-100) material, the response has been determined to be from about 1.1 to 1.4 times greater at low energies than at higher energies (cobalt 60). Although this is not the ideal response and may possibly introduce some error in dose determination, TLD's offer the most reliable method of CT dose measurement.

For CT dose measurement using TLD material, TLD-100 chips ($3 \times 3 \times 1$ mm.) have proved to be most convenient. For calibration the TLD's were irradiated with 3 to 10 rads of cobalt 60 and read out individually. The dosimeters were then grouped according to sensitivity, and the group-adjusted calibration values were used. The TLD's were read out on either a Harshaw 2000B TLD reader or an Eberline TL-5 reader with a low pre-read temperature of 150° C. and a read-out temperature of 240° C. The annealing technique consisted in heating the TLD chips for 1 hour at 400° C. and 24 hours at 80° C.

The CT x-ray beam for most CT units has sufficient penumbra that there is generally a significant difference in radiation dose for a single scan versus multiple scans, with an increment between each scan equal to the slice thickness. For multiple scans the dose pattern along the axis of the subject has radiation dose undulations that differ by as much as 30 to 90 per cent, depending upon the degree of x-ray beam overlap and penumbra. As a result, it is possible to get large differences in radiation dose determination for multiple CT scans depending upon the position of the dosimeter. To avoid this problem, one can obtain the radiation dose profile across a single scan slice using 20 TLD chips in a row. From single dose profiles one can calculate the dose values for multiple scans at any scan increment distance. Construction of a multiple scan dose profile from a single scan dose profile is shown in Figure 7–1.

A convenient method of packaging the TLD chips consists of placing them side by side in a plastic coin envelope and tightly heat-sealing the envelope to

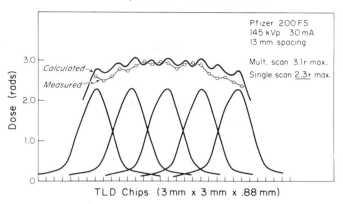

Figure 7–1. Construction of a multiple-scan dose profile from that for a single scan. The single scan dose profiles are spaced so that the peak-to-peak separation equals 13 mm., which is the slice thickness. (From McCullough, E. C., and Payne, J. T.: Patient dose in computed tomography. Radiology, *129*:457–463, 1978. Reproduced by permission.)

maintain a line of TLD's. To insure reproducible CT dose measurements, standard phantoms should be used. For this reason it is recommended that head doses be measured using an 8½-inch diameter by 3-inch thick acrylic cylinder and body doses using an 8-inch by 13-inch elliptical phantom. Single scan doses can be measured at any position "in" or "on" the phantom, provided that TLD insert holes have been drilled in the phantom. Sufficient information can be obtained by measuring the dose at 5 sites: top, bottom, center, and both sides of the phantom. At the time of CT dose measurement, all pertinent CT operating parameters such as kVp, mA, scan time, filtration, slice thickness, pixel size, noise, resolution, and patient bolus must be noted. Multiple scan dose can then be calculated from the single scan data using a designated scan increment distance (generally a distance equal to the slice thickness).

To obtain a representative value of radiation dose at CT x-ray energies, the dose as obtained using the TLD chips calibrated in cobalt rads is divided by a factor of 1.3 to correct for the energy response of the TLD material and the difference in "f" factors for muscle from high to low photon energy. Using this method and taking into account the precision of TLD measurements, it is felt that the CT dose values are probably accurate to within ± 20 per cent, which is sufficient for this purpose. The use of cobalt 60 as the source of TLD calibration was adopted to insure better consistency from institution to institution and because it is generally being used for TLD calibration.

MEASURED CT RADIATION DOSE

Radiation doses have been measured from various CT units, including an EMI Mark I, 5005, and 1005, a Pfizer 200 FS, Delta 50, 50 FS, and 2020, a GE CT 8800, Siemens Somatom 2, and Picker Synerview 600. A typical single scan profile of radiation dose is shown for a Pfizer 200 FS in Figure 7–2. Using the single-scan profiles, multiple scan doses can be obtained. Measured radiation doses for the above units are shown in Tables 7–1 and 7–2. For these units the multiple to single scan dose ratio was between 1.2 for those units with good collimation and slightly less than 2 for less tightly collimated units. On the average, one can generally anticipate the multiple scan dose to be about 1.5 times greater than the single scan dose. As can be seen from Tables 7–1 and

TABLE 7–1. RADIATION DOSE FROM COMMERCIAL CT UNITS

CT UNIT	STUDY	TECHNIQUE				MAX. SURFACE DOSE, IN RADS, SINGLE SCAN
		kVp	mA	Scan Time(s) (secs.)	Scan Angle	
EMI Mark I	head*	120	33	240	180°	2.7
EMI CT 1005	head	120	33	60/240	180°	3.6/12‡
EMI CT 5005	head	140	28	26/73	180°	2.4/9.6‡
	body	140	28	25/73	180°	3.0/12‡
Pfizer 200	head	140	30	27/45	180°	2.0/4.0
	body	140	30	27	180°	2.4
Delta 25	head	130	30	130/185	192°	5.8/11.6§
Delta 50	head	120	30	120	180°	1.8
	body	120**	30	150	180°	1.4
Delta 50FS	head	140	35	17/27	180°	2.3/4.7
	body	140	35	20/36	180°	2.4/4.8
Delta 2020	head	120	100	4	360°	3.4
(Shaped Response)	body	120	100	2	360°	2.0

From McCullough, E. C., and Payne, J. T.: Patient dose in computed tomography. Radiology, *129*:457–463, 1978. Reproduced by permission.

*"Head" = 8½-inch diameter Plexiglas cylinder; "body" = 8 × 13 inch Plexiglas ellipse (except for the Delta 25 scanner in which a head was simulated with an 8 inch diameter water phantom).

‡With two layers of bolus (about 1.5 in.).

§Data from Weinstein, M. A., Duchesneau, P. M., and MacIntyre, W. J.: White and gray matter of the brain differentiated by computed tomography. Radiology, *122*:699–702, 1977.

**With 6.5 mm. Al total filtration option.

TABLE 7–2. RADIATION DOSE FROM OTHER COMMERCIAL CT UNITS

CT UNIT	STUDY	kVp	mAs*	Scan Time(s) (secs.)	Scan Angle	MAX. SURFACE DOSE, IN RADS, SINGLE SCAN
Pfizer 0450 (AS+E)	head	125†	200-500(1000)‡	5(10)	405°	2.0–5.0(10.0)
	body	125†	200-500(1000)	5(10)	405°	2.2–6.0(12.0)
Picker Synerview 600	head	130	330(660)	3.3(6.6)	360°	2.3(4.5)
	body	130	400	3.3	360°	3.5
GE CT/T-7800	head	120	100-300(1152)	4.8(9.6)	360°	0.5–1.5(5.8)
	body	120	100-300(1152)	4.8(9.6)	360°	0.9–2.6(9.2)
GE CT/T-8800	head	120	550(1152)	4.8(9.6)	360°	2.8(5.8)
	body	120	200-300(1152)	4.8(9.6)	360°	1.7–2.6(9.2)
Siemens Somatom 2	head	125	230(460)	5(10)	360°	1.1(2.2)
	body	125	230(460)	5(10)	360°	1.1(2.2)

From McCullough, E. C., and Payne, J. T.: Patient dose in computed tomography. Radiology, *129*:457-463, 1978. Reproduced by permission.

*For pulsed units (mA/pulse) • (pulses/scan) • (sec./pulse).
†With 2 mm. Al plus 0.25 mm. Cu filtration.
‡Typical clinical value(s) followed by maximum possible value in parenthesis.
§Without Synchronous Microbeam Collimator; 1 mm. Al added filtration.

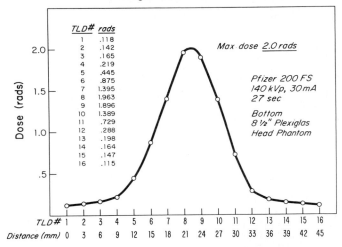

Radiation Dose Profile
Single Scan TLD Profile

TLD#	rads
1	.118
2	.142
3	.165
4	.219
5	.445
6	.875
7	1.395
8	1.963
9	1.896
10	1.389
11	.729
12	.288
13	.198
14	.164
15	.147
16	.115

Max dose 2.0 rads

Pfizer 200 FS
140 kVp, 30 mA
27 sec

Bottom
8 ½" Plexiglas
Head Phantom

Figure 7-2. Measured single scan radiation dose profile at the maximum dose profile at the maximum dose position on the surface of a head phantom using a Pfizer 200 FS CT scanner.

7-2, the doses range from about 2 rads up to 20 rads or more depending upon the quality of the image desired and the various operational parameters of the CT unit. For standard modes of operation, most CT units have a maximum entrance dose of about 2 to 5 rads, with a dose to the center of the patient of about 1 to 2.5 rads.

CT SCANNER DESIGN PARAMETERS AFFECTING RADIATION DOSE

A number of CT scan parameters will affect the radiation dose for any given CT procedure. The most obvious of these would be the x-ray exposure technique, that is, the kVp, mA, time per measurement, and total number of measurements. Reasons for going to high-exposure techniques would be to achieve a reduction in scan noise and improvement in reconstruction accuracy. Reasons for restraints in exposure would be the desire to keep the scan time short; thus, there would be a limitation of the time per data sample and of the available x-ray output per unit time. If one were to make 100,000 measurements (about the number taken by early CT scanners) one at a time at 2 milliseconds per measurement, the data acquisition time alone would be 200 seconds or a little over 3 minutes. If one adds to that the time for mechanical indexing, one arrives at a scan time of 4 to 5 minutes, that of the first EMI CT units. If, however, a group of detectors (10 to 20) is used, the data acquisition time can be reduced to 10 to 20 seconds (EMI 5000). If a larger detector array is employed (200 or more detectors), data acquisition times as short as 1 to 2 seconds can be achieved. In the first two situations, one can generally *not* afford to make more measurements or integrate the transmitted x-ray events for longer time intervals. However, in the last situation, one can *now* make more measurements or integrate for longer times and still have scan times under that of breath holding (10 to 20 seconds). For this reason, the radiation dose from these units may vary from a minimum to a maximum by as much as a factor of 10 or 20, depending upon the x-ray scan technique.

As pointed out previously, CT scanners have been designed to measure small differences in tissue attenuation. One limitation in low-contrast detectability is CT scan noise, which arises to a large extent from the statistical uncertainty of the measurements. A relationship derived by Brooks et al. for the standard deviation of reconstructed CT matrix values is:

$$\sigma(\mu) \, \alpha \left[\frac{B}{W^3 h D_0} \right]^{1/2} \qquad \sigma(\mu) = \text{standard deviation}$$

where μ = linear attenuation coefficient
    B = fractional attenuation of the subject
    W = detector width
    h = slice thickness
    D_0 = maximum entrance dose

From this relationship it can be seen that even CT parameters such as detector width and slice thickness will greatly influence scan noise. Reducing the detector width by 2 requires an increase in entrance dose by a factor of 8 to keep the noise at the same level. Because of ultimate practical limitations in pixel width and slice thickness, low-noise CT scans will generally require higher doses. This assumes that there is no additional smoothing of the projection data or reconstructed image by mathematical methods.

Radiation dose is also influenced by the x-ray focal spot size, collimation, and filtration. Large focal spots (on the order of 2 mm. × 20 mm.) will give rise to a larger penumbra and hence a higher radiation dose for multiple scan sequences. CT units with scan times of 20 seconds or greater generally require oil-cooled continuous output therapy type x-ray tubes with large focal spots. CT units with scan times on the order of 10 seconds or less can use rotating anode diagnostic type x-ray tubes with smaller focal spots (nominal size of 1 to 2 mm.). Based on radiation measurements, it is estimated that the use of small focal spot x-ray tubes can potentially reduce the multiple scan dose by 10 to 40 per cent. One method of reducing this effect in large focal spot units (2 mm. × 20 mm.) is the use of one or more collimator plates or fins placed in the collimator slot. The fins are perpendicular to the long axis of the focal spot and help to "parallelize" the diverging x-rays. The use of such fins in the EMI 5005 and the Pfizer 200 FS units can significantly reduce the overall dose. Multiple to single scan ratios for different CT scanners are shown in Table 7–3.

In order to minimize beam-hardening artifacts, a reasonably heavily filtered x-ray source is advantageous. However, with heavy filtration a large reduction in x-ray incident intensity results and CT scan noise generally increases. For this reason, filtration is generally limited to 3 or 4 mm. of aluminum; however, in certain high output CT units, 0.5 mm. copper filtration has been employed. Use of the copper filter generally reduces the beam-hardening artifacts and lowers the patient dose. This type of filter is currently used in the Siemens Somatom 2 unit.

Detector design also influences the radiation dose to the patient. To minimize patient dose, the detector should have a high photon capture ratio. For multiple detector arrays this means that the dead space between detectors must be kept at a minimum. From this standpoint, rotational multiple array detectors (such as xenon chambers or CsI minicrystal arrays) offer an advantage and have a high photon capture ratio. However, the detector conversion

TABLE 7–3. MULTIPLE TO SINGLE SCAN RADIATION DOSE RATIOS FOR VARIOUS CT UNITS

CT UNIT	SLICE THICKNESS (MM.)*	SLICES PER SCAN	TABLE INCREMENT	MULTIPLE/SINGLE RATIO
Rotate/translate				
EMI				
Mark I	10.5	2	20	1.7†
1005	10.3	2	20	1.8
5005	13.2	1	13	1.9
Pfizer				
200 FS	9.0	1	10	1.6
Ohio-Nuclear				
50 FS2	10.4	2	20	1.7
25	13.0	2	26	1.5
Rotary				
General Electric				
7800/8800	10.4	1	10	1.2
Ohio-Nuclear				
2020 (Shaped Response)	10.0	1	10	1.4
Siemens				
Somatom 2	10.0	1	10	1.6
Pfizer AS+E				
0450	10.0	1	10	1.8
Picker Synerview				
600	10.0	1	10	1.2

From McCullough, E. C., and Payne, J. T.: Patient dose in computed tomography. Radiology, *129*:457–463, 1978. Reproduced by permission.

*FWHM at isocenter.

†Estimated uncertainty due to 3 mm. sampling of single scan profile is ±0.1.

efficiency for captured photons should also be high. This latter condition favors scintillation detectors such as NaI, BGO (bismuth germinate), CsI, and to a lesser extent CaF_2. (It takes about a 2-inch path length of CaF_2 for a 95 per cent absorption.) Stationary array detector systems with 600 or more BGO detectors are potentially capable of having both high capture ratios and high conversion efficiencies if high spatial resolution limitations are relaxed. For this geometry (Pfizer AS+E scanner) the detector length is 5 to 6 mm. with 600 detectors spaced evenly in a stationary ring of about 1.5 m. diameter. However, to obtain spatial resolution approaching 1 mm. or better requires the masking off of the detector so that the detected x-ray beam is narrower. This gives rise to a high radiation dose due to significant collimation losses. If, however, spatial resolution on the order of about 2 mm. is accepted, this design offers one of the best capture and conversion efficiencies. The detection efficiency for third and fourth generation CT scanners is shown in Table 7–4.

Finally, patient dose will be influenced by the source-to-patient distance

TABLE 7–4. EFFICIENCY OF THIRD- AND FOURTH-GENERATION CT UNITS

GENERATION	DETECTORS	CAPTURE RATIO (%)	DETECTOR EFFICIENCY (%)	DETECTION EFFICIENCY (%)
Third	Rotary	90	60 (Xenon)	54
		90	98 (CsI)	88
Fourth	Fixed	50	98 (BGO, CsI)*	49
		90	98 (BGO, CsI)†	88

From McCullough, E. C., and Payne, J. T.: Patient dose in computer tomography. Radiology, *129*:457–463, 1978. Reproduced by permission.

*Xenon is not used in fixed-detector geometry, since x-rays do not always enter perpendicular to the front surface of the detector.

†Stationary array detector rings containing 1200 or more detectors.

and CT scanner motion. Dedicated head scanners and stationary array units with the source inside the detector ring will have closer source-to-patient distances and higher patient doses than translate-rotate or rotational moving detector array body CT units. In addition, CT scanner motion (i.e., 180° versus 360° rotation) will influence the distribution of the dose. For 180° translate-rotate units, the dose is a maximum on one side, whereas for a 360° unit the dose is more uniformly spread over the surface of the patient. However, for the present units of both types (180° versus 360°), the maximum surface doses for reasonably similar image quality are not drastically different.

CT DOSE IN COMPARISON TO OTHER DIAGNOSTIC RADIOLOGY DOSES

Finally, it is important to view the radiation exposure from CT scanning in light of the exposure from other conventional x-ray procedures. From the previous discussion, nominal CT surface doses are on on the order of 2 to 5 rads per study for the area scanned. For a single x-ray film the entrance dose can range from as low as 20 millirads to slightly under a rad, depending upon the area irradiated. Typical x-ray dose values are indicated in Table 7–5. As can be seen, the doses range from as low as a fraction of a rad to as high as 10 rads for a single exam. In fact, in many special procedures involving angiography or pneumoencephalography the dose can be as high as 40 rads or more. From this standpoint the radiation dose from a CT scan is low. Thus, the CT radiation dose is in line with that of most conventional x-ray procedures and lower than most special procedures. Because the radiation dose is not negligible, CT scanning is not a screening procedure from this standpoint. Discretion should therefore be used in ordering patient CT exams, and they should be administered only when clinically warranted.

RESEARCH FINDINGS

Several CT radiation dose studies will be discussed with respect to the results obtained. Those interested in methodology or other details should refer to the original articles. One of the first dose studies in clinical CT was reported by Perry and Bridges (1973). They measured CT doses in the range of 1 to 2.5 rads to the head for a series of scans and a gonadal dose of less than 0.1 mrad from an EMI head unit. Doses outside of the primary beam have been measured by McCullough for an EMI CT 5005 and are shown in Table 7–6.

Bhave et al. (1977) conducted a study in which they investigated the scattered radiation dose to the eyes, thyroids, and gonads in infants and children during CT scanning of the head. An EMI scanner was used and TLD

TABLE 7–5.   CONVENTIONAL RADIOLOGY DOSES

EXAMINATION	SURFACE RADIATION DOSE (RADS)
Skull series (4 films)	0.5
Angiogram (11 films/biplane)	10.0
Pneumo (18 films)	3.0
Abdomen (1 film)	0.2
Liver scan (3mCi Tc-S)	1.0
Brain scan (15mCi Tc)	0.2 Brain
	1.5 GI

TABLE 7–6. ORGAN DOSES DUE TO SECONDARY RADIATIONS IN A CT SCANNER*

SCAN SITE	DOSE SITE	INTERNAL† SCATTER	LEAD APRON‡ (ABOVE/BELOW)	DOSE PER SCAN (MRADS)
head§	ovaries§	+	–/–	0.066
head	ovaries	–	–/–	0.050
head	ovaries	–	+/–	0.026
head	ovaries	–	+/+	0.006
thorax§	ovaries	+	–/–	0.38
thorax	ovaries	–	–/–	0.28
thorax	ovaries	–	+/–	0.11
thorax	ovaries	–	+/+	0.035

Scan Site	Dose Site	Dose per scan (mrads)
head	eyes§	120
head	thyroid§	10
head	ovaries	0.066/0.022
thorax	eyes	10
thorax	thyroid	30
thorax	ovaries	0.38/0.14**

From McCullough, E. C., and Payne, J. T.: Patient dose in computed tomography. Radiology, *129*:457–463, 1978. Reproduced by permission.

*All data from EMI CT 5005, 140 kVp, 28 mA, single scan, "normal" (25 sec.) scan time and with bolus. Measured using an Alderson "sectioned" phantom.

†+ no lead plate between sections 16 and 17.

‡0.25 mm. Pb equivalent; + = apron present.

§Head, section 1; thorax, section 15; ovaries, section 28; eyes, section 3; thyroid, section 7. Each phantom section is approximately 1 inch thick.

**Without/with lead aprons above and below.

dosimeters were positioned near the left eye, over the thyroid, and on the lower abdomen in close proximity to the gonads. They reported an average skin dose of 1.3 rads per scan and doses to the eyes, thyroid, and gonads to be 850 mrads, 310 mrads, and 30 mrads, respectively.

Pediatric CT doses were investigated by Brasch et al. (1978). Two phantoms were constructed to approximate a 10-year-old child and a 6-month-old infant. TLD dosimeters were used to determine surface and internal radiation doses from several body CT scanners. They found the range of CT doses to be from 0.4 to 5.6 rads for pediatric body scans.

DOSE-REDUCTION METHODS

Because radiation dose to patients even at low levels carries with it a possible genetic or carcinogenic risk, radiation dose from CT scans should be kept as low as possible. Radiation dose may be kept at a minimum in CT scanning by employing improved collimation with small focal spot x-ray tubes that will reduce penumbra and thus reduce the "overlap" dose for adjacent cuts of a multiple scan CT series. This can lower the total dose by as much as 50 to 60 per cent. If high-resolution, low-noise scans are not really required, one can reduce the number of views and x-ray output and significantly lower patient dose by a factor of two or more. Maximizing filtration will harden the x-ray beam and reduce the entrance exposure to the patient. Gonadal shielding, where possible, should still be employed. However, the gonadal shield will probably introduce artifacts into the scan, so such shielding may not always be practical. Reducing the total number of slices taken would also be helpful, and if possible one should avoid re-scanning over the same area. Shorter scans will reduce motion artifacts and thus lower the repeat rate.

CT / 7

SUMMARY/REFERENCES/BIBLIOGRAPHY/REVIEW QUESTIONS

Summary

1. Dose values in CT scanning will depend primarily on four factors: (a) single scan image quality, (b) detection efficiency, (c) the details of the scan motion, and (d) multiple scan geometry. Lower limits on patient dosage in CT scanning are intimately related to requirements for single scan image quality (noise, resolution, and slice thickness).

2. Improvements in image quality such as narrower slice thickness, increased resolution (e.g., smaller pixel width), or increased contrast resolution (i.e., lower scan noise) usually require increased patient dose.

3. Values of patient dosage from clinically used CT scan techniques range from 2 to 10 rads/study (5 or more slices) but for both rotate-translate and pure rotary motion scanners larger dose/study values are possible. It is not possible to make a blanket statement about whether any scan "generation" offers an equivalent or higher quality image for less dosage to the patient.

4. Secondary radiation dosages to the patient appear to be small but in certain instances can be reduced by lead aprons (at least 0.25 mm. Pb equivalency) above and below the patient.

5. Dose values near the CT scanner are about 1 to 2 mrads/scan at 1 meter from the scan circle.

6. Dose reduction methods in CT relate to collimation, x-ray focal spot size, filtration, number of data points taken, pixel size, and shielding.

References

Agarwal, S. K., Friesen, E. J., Bhaduri, D., and Courlas, G.: Dose distribution from a Delta-25 head scanner. Med. Phys., 6(4):302–304, July/Aug., 1979.

Baker, H. L., Campbell, J. H., Houser, O. W., et al.: Early experience with the EMI scanner for study of the brain. Radiology, 116:327–333, 1975.

Bhave, D. G., et al.: Scattered radiation doses to infants and children during EMI head scans. Radiology, 124:379–380, 1977.

Brasch, R. C., Boyd, D. P., and Gooding, C. A.: Computed tomographic scanning in children. Comparison of radiation dose and resolving power of commercial CT scanners. Am. J. Roentgenol., 131:95–101, 1978.

Cronin, M. P.: X-ray dose reduction in computed tomography. Appl. Radiol., 6:111–115, Jan./Feb., 1977.

Ewen, K., Fischer, P. G., and Fiebach, B. J. O.: Exposure to useful and scattered radiation in computer tomography. Electromedica, 1:7–8, 1977.

Gross, G., and McCullough, E. C.: Exposure values around an x-ray scanning transaxial tomograph (EMI scanner). Med. Phys., 2(5):282–283, Sept./Oct., 1975.

Gross, G., and McCullough, E. C.: Radiation protection requirements for a whole-body CT scanner. Radiology, 122:825–826, 1977.

Isherwood, I., et al.: Radiation dose to the eyes of the patient during neuroradiological investigations. Neuroradiology, 10:137–141, 1975.

Jucius, R. A., and Kambic, G. X.: Radiation dosimetry in computed tomography (CT). Proceedings of the Society of Photo-Optical Instrumentation Engineers, "Application of Optical Instrumentation in Medicine," 127:286–295, 1977.

Maue-Dickson, W., Trefler, M., and Dickson, D. R.: Comparison of dosimetry and image quality in computed and conventional tomography. Radiology, 131:509–514, 1979.

McCullough, E. C., and Payne, J. T.: Patient dose in computed tomography. Radiology, *129*:457–463, 1978.

Perry, B. J., and Bridges, C.: Computerized transverse axial scanning (tomography). Part 3. Radiation dose considerations. Br. J. Radiol., *46*:1048–1051, 1973.

Raeside, D. E., Anderson, D. W., and Alloway, D. C.: A study of the dose to the thyroid and the eye in computed tomography of the brain. Radiology, *129*:814–815, 1978.

Shrivastava, P. N., Lynn, S. L., and Ting, J. Y.: Exposures to patient and personnel in computed axial tomography. Radiology, *125*:411–415, 1977.

Sorensen, J. A.: Evaluation of CT parameters. Med. Phys., *6*:68–69, 1979.

Weinstein, M. D., Duchesneau, P. M., and MacIntyre, W. J.: White and gray matter of the brain differentiated by computed tomography. Radiology, *122*:699–702, 1977.

Whitmore, R. C., et al.: Radiation dose in neurological computed tomographic scanning. Radiol. Tech., *51*:21–26, 1979.

Bibliography

Bhave, D. C., et al.: Scattered radiation doses to infants and children during EMI head scans. Radiology, *124*:379–380, 1977.

Gross, G., and McCullough, E. C.: Radiation protection requirements for a whole-body CT scanner. Radiology, *122*:825–826, 1977.

Maue-Dickson, W., Trefler, M., and Dickson, D. R.: Comparison of dosimetry and image quality in computed and conventional tomography. Radiology, *131*:509–514, 1979.

Shrivastava, P. N., Lynn, S. L., and Ting, J. Y.: Exposures to patient and personnel in computed axial tomography. Radiology, *125*:411–415, 1977.

Whitmore, R. C., et al.: Radiation dose in neurological computed tomographic scanning. Radiol. Tech., *51*:21–26, 1979.

Review Questions

1. Dose in CT is important, since it yields information relating to:
   (a) Evaluation of a benefit/risk ratio.
   (b) The patient's medical condition.
   (c) Bioeffects of high energy x-rays.
   (d) Screening patients of reproductive age for intracranial and intra-abdominal lesions.

2. Which of the following influences dose in conventional x-ray imaging?
   (a) kVp and filtration.
   (b) Voltage waveform and milliampere seconds.
   (c) Distance from focal spot to object being radiographed and the x-ray field size.
   (d) All of the above.

3. Factors that influence dose in CT are:
   (a) Focal spot size and kVp.
   (b) X-ray source-to-detector distance and the duration of the exposure.
   (c) Filtration, milliamperage, and the number of scans taken.
   (d) All of the above.

4. The way in which the x-ray beam is distributed on the patient during a single CT scan is called:
   (a) Sensitivity profile.
   (b) Alignment profile.
   (c) Collimation profile.
   (d) Dose profile.

5. Which is *not* a method to reduce dose in CT?
   (a) Use of faster photographic films to record the anatomy.
   (b) Improved collimation to reduce penumbra.

(c) Maximizing filtration.
(d) Reducing the number of scans and hence data collection.

6. The patient dose from a CT exam is generally about:
   (a) 1 to 2 millirads.
   (b) 2 to 5 kilorads.
   (c) 10 to 20 rads.
   (d) 2 to 5 rads.

7. Generally, the most accurate way to measure CT dose is with:
   (a) Film.
   (b) Ionization chamber.
   (c) TLD's.
   (d) GM counter.

8. The radiation dose from third-generation scanners is significantly less than from fourth-generation units.
   (a) Yes
   (b) No
   (c) Has not been determined

9. The radiation dose from CT scanning is significantly less than from conventional x-ray studies.
   (a) Yes
   (b) No
   (c) Has not been determined

10. As slice thickness is changed from 10 mm. to 5 mm., the radiation dose must be _____ by_____ in order to maintain the same noise value.
    (a) increased, 2x
    (b) decreased, 2x
    (c) increased, 4x
    (d) decreased, 4x

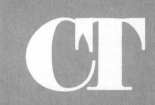

CHAPTER 8

SOME CLINICAL CONSIDERATIONS

The computerized tomograph can assist in the diagnosis of pathologies in almost every part of the body including the brain, structures of the face, spinal cord, bones, lungs, heart, organs of the abdomen and pelvis and extremities.

ROBERT S. LEDLEY (1977)

The purpose of this chapter is to present an overview of some clinical aspects of CT, such as patient positioning, preparation, scanning technical factors, indications, and the use of contrast media. The reader must realize that scanning protocols for CT will differ from place to place, and therefore exact details will not be discussed here. The more ambitious student should refer to several texts on clinical CT (Felson, 1977; Norman et al., 1977; Hanaway et al., 1977; Bories, 1978; Love, 1979; Sodee, 1979) for a more comprehensive coverage of clinical applications.

CT OF THE HEAD

CLINICAL EFFICACY

The term *clinical efficacy* refers to the acquisition of relevant information that can be used to provide a direct improvement in total patient care and management (Manfredi, 1979). Today, CT of the head is a well-established technique in the investigation and detection of intracranial disorders. These disorders include meningiomas, gliomas and metastases, intraorbital lesions, posterior fossa tumors, cerebral infarction, aneurysms and arteriovenous malformations, hypertensive intracranial hemorrhage, head trauma, abscesses, calcifications, hydrocephalus, and cerebral atrophy.

In children, the usefulness of CT in the evaluation of intracranial disorders has also been well documented. Naidich and Kricheff (1976), for example, have reported that CT is a safe, rapid, and reliable tool in evaluating hydrocephalus, trauma, neoplasms (astrocytoma, medulloblastoma, brain stem glioma, craniopharyngioma, pinealoma) and cerebrovascular disease in the pediatric patient.

In the detection of orbital lesions and demonstration of the globe, optic nerve, periglobal fat, and extraocular muscles, CT has been reported to be a useful new technique (Lampert et al., 1974; Chu, 1977).

In its present form, CT is replacing such procedures as cerebral angiography, pneumoencephalography, ventriculography, and in some cases routine skull series.

Finally, CT of the head has been identified as a most efficacious procedure because of its noninvasiveness and its ability to provide information with great speed and accuracy.

INDICATIONS

Several indications have already been identified in the foregoing discussion. CT of the head can also be useful in providing information relating to:

a. The general size and shape of structures or masses in the brain.

b. The relationships of these masses or structures to other regions in the head.

c. Effects of trauma.

d. The detection of metastases.

e. The benign or malignant nature of abnormalities.

f. Space-occupying lesions.

g. Therapy planning and determination of prognosis.

PATIENT PREPARATION

Patient preparation for head studies may differ from hospital to hospital; however, there are a number of key elements inherent in good preparation.

First, there is the communication element. This involves an explanation of the examination to the patient, which can be done by a physician, nurse, or technologist. The radiologist and CT technologist should reassure the patient with a further explanation or clarification of the scanning process. Explanations should be brief and simple. A suggested sequence of points in explaining a CT examination to a patient is given in Table 8–1.

The element of risk should also be mentioned to the patient in examinations in which contrast material is used. In this case, a history of allergies should be recorded so that the staff may be fully prepared for patient reactions to contrast media.

TABLE 8–1. SUGGESTED SEQUENCE OF POINTS IN EXPLAINING A CT EXAMINATION TO A PATIENT

—Explain the term *CT* briefly, stressing the use of a computer to produce the picture.
—Describe the length of the procedure.
—Briefly explain the equipment (e.g., gantry, table, computers, etc.).
—Explain positioning and the direction of movement through the gantry during the examination.
—Emphasize the importance of remaining perfectly immobile during the exposure (audible signal), stressing the production of artifacts with motion.
—Give breathing instructions before the exposure.
—Explain the use of contrast material and reason for use.
—Give the patient opportunity to ask questions before scanning commences.

Secondly, hair pins and any other metallic (or other) structures (used for cosmetic purposes) should be removed from the patient's head, as these can produce streak artifacts on the CT image.

In some cases, it may be necessary to use sedation such as intravenous diazepam (Valium) for adults and chloral hydrate for children; general anesthesia may be necessary in situations in which patients are agitated and uncooperative.

Sedation protocols will differ from department to department; for example, Anderson and Osborn (1977) report the use of a mixture of meperidine, chlorpromazine, and promethazine ("cardiac cocktail") in scanning pediatric patients. This results in good CT images with "no important complications" and several advantages, including low costs, nonhospitalization of patients, and "random scheduling" of patients.

PATIENT POSITIONING AND SCANNING

Positioning the head for a CT examination will vary depending upon the structures to be examined. The scans are usually taken in relationship to the *infraorbitomeatal line* (Reid's base line — a line drawn from the infraorbital margin to the external auditory meatus), which is used as a base line in determining various degrees of angulation.

In positioning the head, Reid's base line is placed perpendicular to the horizontal plane so that the patient's head is in a "relaxed" position. It is for this reason that the use of this base line became common. It is interesting to note here that other base lines, for example, the cantomeatal line (Huckman et al., 1977), have been used in CT of the head.

Scans are usually taken with the following angulations:

1. 0° (Fig. 8–1*A*). In this case, the scan is parallel to Reid's base line. This degree of angulation would be used to examine details of orbits, sella turcica, and suprasellar area (Lin, 1976).

2. 20 to 25° (Fig. 8–1*B*). This range of angulation would be used to examine posterior fossa structures (Lin, 1976).

Having determined the angulation to be used, the patient is placed supine on the scanning couch, and the head is inserted into the aperture of the gantry for the scanning sequence. This sequence will involve a number of scans to cover the area from the base of the skull to the vertex. The slice thickness selected will vary from department to department but will generally be set at 10 mm. for standard scans. Figure 8–2 (*A* through *F*) illustrates a scan sequence from base to vertex using 0° angulation.

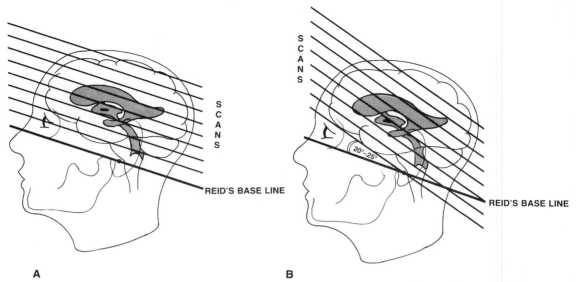

A   **B**

Figure 8–1.   Scan positions for various degrees of angulation using Reid's base line as a reference.

In Figure 8–3, some aspects of patient positioning for CT of the head are shown, while Figure 8–4 shows several clinical images demonstrating some anatomical areas of interest.

During positioning, the patient should be handled so as to avoid unnecessary pain or anxiety. This is especially important in trauma and pediatric patients. Patient comfort is of primary importance during the scanning sequence. This can be accomplished through the use of immobilization devices, pads, sheets, etc. With infants it is especially important to use blankets and heating pads to maintain body temperature (Naidich and Kricheff, 1976).

During the scanning sequence, the patient must be observed carefully, particularly if contrast material has been administered. After scanning is terminated, the patient should be allowed to sit up on the table (for a brief moment) before stepping off. (Obviously, this does not apply to "stretcher patients.")

CONTRAST ENHANCEMENT

A number of workers (Gado, 1976; Huckman, 1975; Kramer et al., 1975) have proved the usefulness of contrast media in CT of the brain. This technique was already identified in Chapter 6 on image quality. In review, the purpose of contrast media in head CT scanning is to improve visualization of certain structures, especially intravascular blood (Huckman et al., 1977) and to assist in discriminating between neoplastic and non-neoplastic lesions in ambiguous situations (New, 1975).

Text continued on page 169

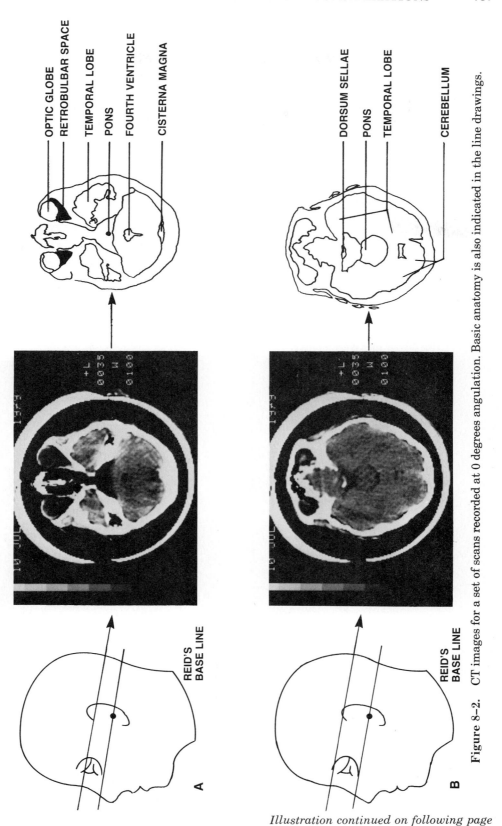

Figure 8-2. CT images for a set of scans recorded at 0 degrees angulation. Basic anatomy is also indicated in the line drawings.

Illustration continued on following page

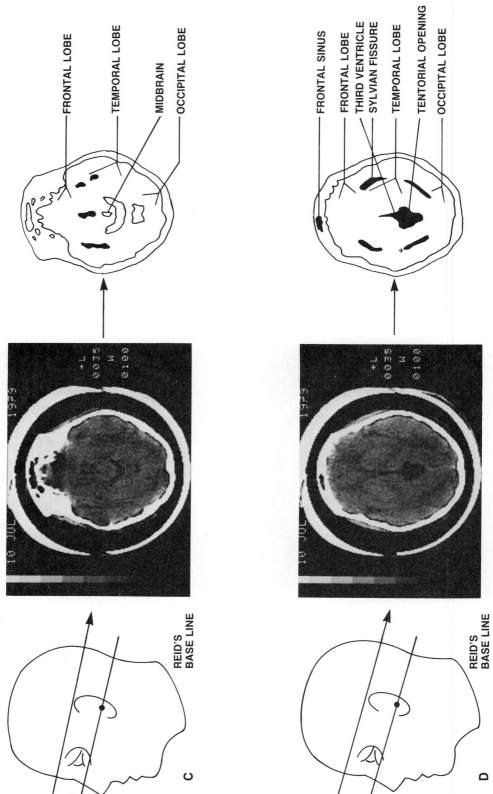

Figure 8–2C,D *Continued*

Illustration continued on opposite page

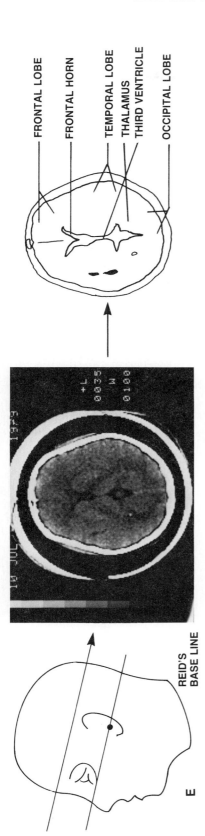

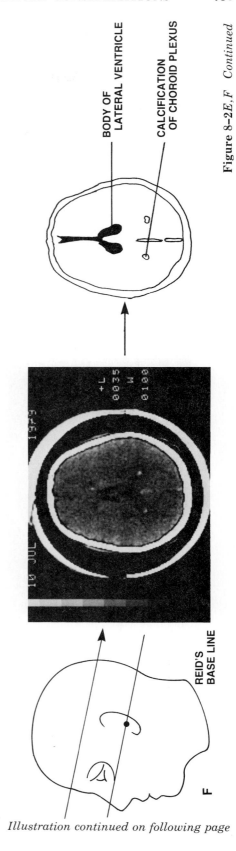

Figure 8–2E,F Continued

Illustration continued on following page

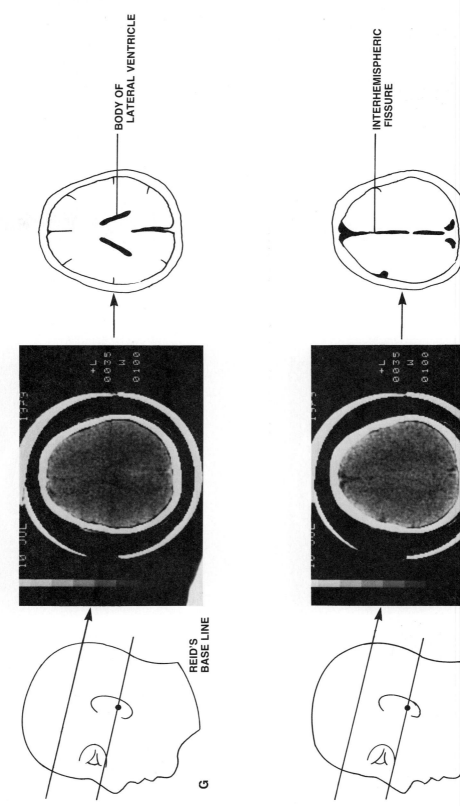

BODY OF LATERAL VENTRICLE

INTERHEMISPHERIC FISSURE

REID'S BASE LINE

REID'S BASE LINE

G

H

Figure 8-2G,H Continued

Illustration continued on opposite page

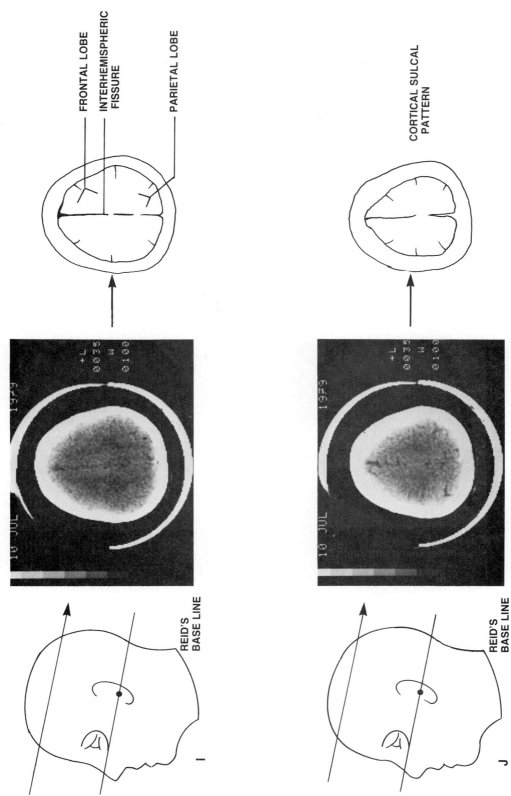

FRONTAL LOBE
INTERHEMISPHERIC FISSURE
PARIETAL LOBE

CORTICAL SULCAL PATTERN

REID'S BASE LINE

REID'S BASE LINE

Figure 8-2I,J Continued

Illustration continued on following page

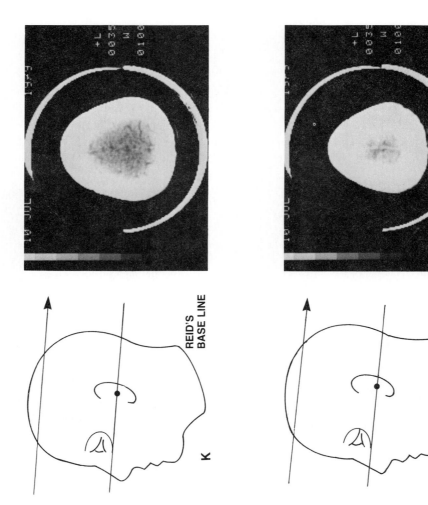

Figure 8–2K,L *Continued*

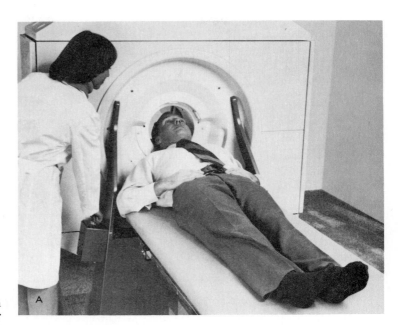

Figure 8–3. Some steps in positioning of the patient for CT of the head. (Photographs provided by the Department of Professional Education, EMI Medical, Inc., Northbrook, Illinois.)

Illustration continued on following page

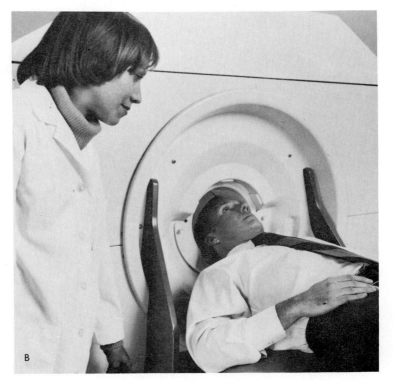

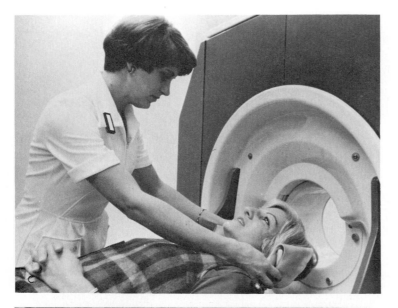

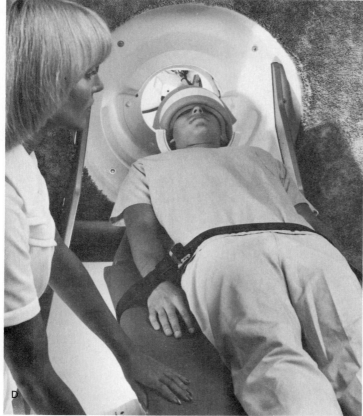

Figure 8–3C,D *Continued*

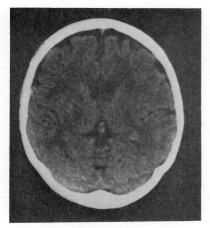

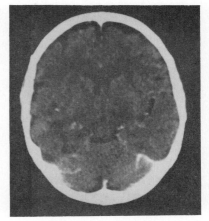

A, CT scan of the head. Lateral ventricles and superior aspect of the vermis are well visualized. Note the excellent delineation of central white from gray matter. Bone-brain interface is beautifully demonstrated.

B, CT scan of the head. The corpora quadrigemina and quadrigeminal cistern are well visualized. Branches of the middle cerebral artery can be seen in the Sylvian fissure. Note the excellent separation of central white from gray matter.

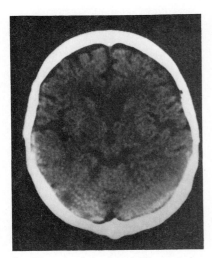

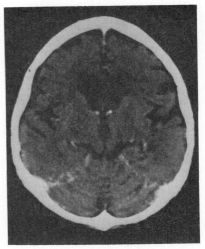

C, CT scan of the head. The anterior and posterior limbs of the internal capsule are well demonstrated bilaterally. Note the central cortical atrophy.

D, CT scan of the head. The ventricles are slightly enlarged and there is cortical atrophy. Note the excellent bone-brain interface.

Figure 8–4. A set of clinical images of the head demonstrating some interesting cases. (Courtesy of Pfizer/American Science and Engineering.)

Illustration continued on following page

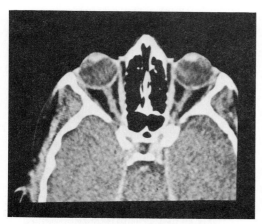

E, In this scan of the orbit, the optic nerves, extraocular muscles, and the lenses are easily seen. As an additional indication of high spatial resolution, one can see the ophthalmic arteries crossing both optic nerves.

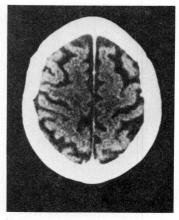

F, This scan shows a view of the vertex with moderately enlarged sulci and interhemispheric fissure.

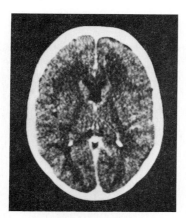

G, The falx cerebri and choroid plexi are contrast-enhanced in this image. Of particular note is the clear visualization of the caudate nucleus and internal capsule which result from excellent contrast resolution.

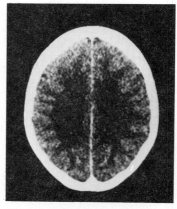

H, High-contrast resolution clearly differentiates white and gray matter in this head scan. The contrast-enhanced midline sutures are clearly seen.

Figure 8–4E,F,G,H   Continued

Illustration continued on opposite page

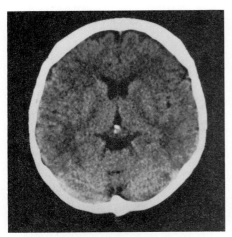

I, CT scan of the head. The quadrigeminal cistern and corpora quadrigemina are beautifully demonstrated. Note the excellent separation of central white from peripheral gray matter.

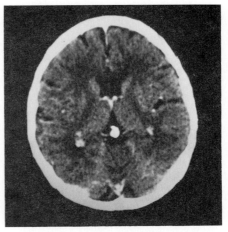

J, CT scan of the head. The caudate nuclei and anterior and posterior limbs of the internal capsule are well visualized. Note the anterior segments of the internal cerebral veins.

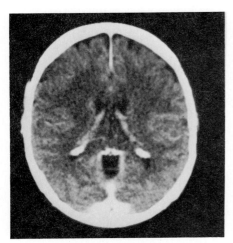

K, CT scan of the head. The choroid plexus is well demonstrated. Note the excellent separation of central white and gray matter.

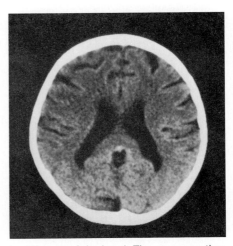

L, CT scan of the head. The upper portion of the ventricles and supracerebellar cistern are well demonstrated. Note the excellent separation of central white and peripheral gray matter.

Figure 8–4*I,J,K,L*   *Continued*

Illustration continued on following page

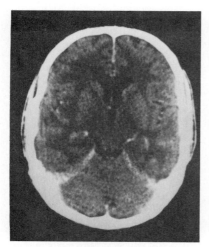

M, CT scan of the head. The internal cerebral veins, caudate nuclei, and anterior and posterior limbs of the internal capsule are well demonstrated.

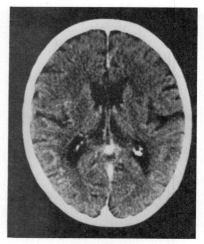

N, CT scan of the head. The caudate nuclei and anterior and posterior limbs of the internal capsule are well demonstrated. Note the excellent separation of central white from gray matter.

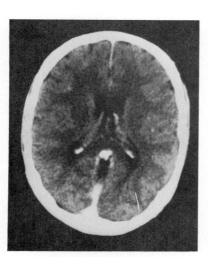

O, CT scan of the head. The lateral ventricles and choroid plexus are well demonstrated. The centrum semiovale is beautifully shown.

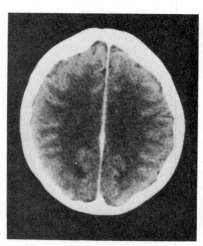

P, CT scan of the head. The centrum semiovale is beautifully demonstrated. The superior aspects of the lateral ventricles can be seen. Note the excellent bone-brain interface.

Figure 8–4*M,N,O,P Continued*

The method of administration (bolus or drip infusion) and the amount of contrast (iodinated contrast) used will depend on the radiologist and the patient's clinical data. Scanning usually commences after some contrast has been introduced and continued (infusion) during the scanning process so that constant blood-iodine levels are maintained (Lin, 1976).

Recently, Norman et al. (1978) reported that in a study of malignant gliomas a dose of 28 to 42 grams of iodine has been found to be optimal for acceptable diagnostic results. They also stated that this optimal dose means that a 10-minute blood-iodine level of 100 mg./100 ml. is needed for acceptable contrast enhancement of tumors.

CT OF THE BODY

CT of the body includes scanning the *neck, thorax, abdomen, pelvis,* and *upper and lower extremities.*

EFFICACY

CT of the body now receives widespread acceptance since it has been well established in demonstrating a number of specific conditions (Table 8–2). In some cases, it has been regarded as the most definitive procedure (Skalnik, 1977). Although controversies still sometimes surface concerning the efficacy of body CT, it still continues to progress at a rapid rate, generating an enormous amount of information that is not within the realm of this chapter.

INDICATIONS

As CT body investigations continue, more and more indications are becoming apparent. In 1979, the Society for Body Computed Tomography published a new set of indications for body CT in the *American Journal of Roentgenology.* These indications are given in the Appendix.

PATIENT PREPARATION, POSITIONING, AND SCANNING

It is important to realize that patient preparation, positioning, and details of the scanning sequence for body CT will differ somewhat from department to department. Such differences will depend on a number of factors, such as the patient's clinical data, the specific organ to be examined, the scanning capabilities of the CT unit, the radiologist's preference, and so on.

Good bowel preparation is of utmost importance in scanning abdominal regions, as old barium residues, for example, could result in a degradation of image quality (Churchill et al., 1979).

Positioning of the patient is a simple procedure and usually involves placing him/her in the supine position (although prone and decubitus positions are not uncommon) for most studies of chest, abdomen, pelvis, and extremities.

TABLE 8–2. SOME PROCESSES DEMONSTRATED BY BODY CT

Liver and biliary system
Primary and metastic tumors
Nodular hyperplasia with cirrhosis
Fatty infiltration
Hemochromatosis
Cholangitis
Abscess
Hematoma
Congenital anomalies (e.g.,
    choledochal cyst, polycystic
    diseases, simple cyst)
Dilated bile ducts

Gallbladder
Enlarged gallbladder
Opaque stones

Spleen
Cysts
Infarcts
Sharply defined tumors

Pancreas
Calcifications of chronic pancreatitis
Pseudocysts
Tumors that alter contour or size of
    pancreas

Kidneys and adrenals
Tumors
Cysts
Hemangiomyolipomas
Hydronephrosis
Urinomas
Renal cortical atrophy
Adjacent but separate masses
Status of renal transplant
Adrenal tumor and cysts
Neuroblastoma

Retroperitoneum
Sarcomas
Lymphomas
Metastatic tumors
Fibrosis
Abscess
Hematoma
Cysts
Congenital anomalies
Aortic aneurysm (noncalcified or
    calcified)
Leaking aneurysm

Spine
Metastatic disease and primary tumor
Sequelae of trauma
    Encroachment of spinal canal
    Retroperitoneal hematoma
Congenital anomalies
    (meningocele, dermoid,
        diastematomyelia)
Osteopenia, hematologic disorder
    Paget's disease

Pelvis
Primary and metastatic tumors
Bone destruction
Abscess and inflammatory disease
Hematoma
Congenital anomalies

Extremities
Tumor (soft tissue and bone)
Infection
Hematoma

Chest
Diseases of the mediastinum, chest
    wall, pleura, and pulmonary
    parenchyma
Tumors (total extent)
Complicated inflammatory diseases,
    abscess
Pleural effusion (loculated)

Head and neck
Intracranial, intraorbital, or soft-
    tissue extension of tumors of skull
    base, sinuses, and nasopharynx
Complicated inflammatory disease
Sequelae of trauma
    Intracranial epidural and
        subdural hematoma
    Depressed fractures of skull,
        orbit, and facial bones
Cervical spine fractures
Congenital anomalies

Lymphoma
Enlargement of retroperitoneal
    nodes, especially near hilar areas of
    kidneys, spleen, and liver
Enlargement of intraperitoneal
    nodes
Involvement of discrete areas of liver,
    spleen, and bone and of
    subcutaneous tissue or muscle
    mass

From Carter, B.L., and Ignatow, S.G.: Computed body tomography. How useful is it? Postgrad. Med., *63*:66–80, 1978. Reproduced by permission.

In positioning for body CT, the technologist must adhere to the scanning protocols set up by the radiologist in charge of CT scanning. These scanning protocols give information regarding patient position, the use of external landmarks, the use of contrast media, radiographic factors, and the thickness of the slice to be used. An excellent discussion of scanning protocols for body CT (an example of which is given in Table 8–3) is found in a paper by Kirkpatrick et al. (1978).

TABLE 8-3. AN EXAMPLE OF CT SCANNING PROTOCOLS FOR SEVERAL BODY REGIONS

	PANCREAS	LIVER	JAUNDICE	RETROPERITO-NEUM	PELVIS	THORAX Thymoma	THORAX Pulmonary Mass
Landmark:							
Superior	Xiphoid	3 cm. above xiphoid	Xiphoid	Aortic hiatus	Iliac crest	Sternal notch	Sternal notch
Inferior	Uncinate process	Pericolic gutter	Pericolic gutter	Iliac crest	Symphysis	Carina	Dome of liver
Spacing (mm.)	15	15	15	20	20	15	15
Contrast:							
Oral	Yes	Yes	Yes	Yes	Yes	No	Occasionally
Intravenous	Occasionally	Yes	Occasionally	No	Yes	No	No
Spasmolytic agent	Yes	No	Yes	Yes	No	No	No
Additional techniques	Decubitus, delayed sections, intravenous contrast, 8 mm. collimator	Spasmolytic agent, decubitus	Intravenous contrast, decubitus	Delayed sections	Hydration, spasmolytic agent	Intravenous contrast	Intravenous contrast

From Kirkpatrick, R.H., et al.: Scanning techniques in computed body tomography. Am. J. Roentgenol. *130*:1069–1075, 1978. Reproduced by permission.

Once positioning is accomplished, the area to be scanned is inserted into the gantry aperture and the patient is again instructed to remain perfectly immobile during scanning.

In some situations, preliminary scout views (pre-scan localization) may be used to determine the exact levels of the scanning sequence. This will be discussed later in the chapter.

Figure 8–5 shows patient transfer and positioning for a body scan, while Figure 8–6 illustrates typical scan sequences for the neck, thorax, abdomen, and pelvis. In Figure 8–7 a number of clinical images for body CT are shown. The reader should refer to any CT cross-sectional anatomy text (Meschan, 1978, for example) for identification of the important structures.

Contrast Media

The use of contrast agents is sometimes essential in body CT, "especially when initial plain scan sequences fail to demonstrate a suspected abnormality or further clarification of a demonstrated abnormality is required" (Kirkpatrick et al., 1978).

A number of contrast materials have been used. These include barium and meglumine diatrizoate (Gastrografin — Squibb). Intravenous contrast media are also used (Stephens et al., 1976; Kirkpatrick et al., 1978). These may be administered either by bolus or by the infusion method. Contrast may also be administered orally (Ruijs, 1979) or through the rectum (Churchill et al., 1979).

Other techniques that aid in visualization of certain structures include the use of a tampon in the vagina to outline that structure and carbon dioxide for demonstrating bladder carcinoma (Seidelman, 1977).

Technical Factors

The factors that are considered technical in CT not only refer to radiographic exposure factors but also include the selection of the appropriate collimator, window width, and window level settings.

The most commonly available collimators are the 8 mm., 10 mm., and 13 mm. ones. The selection of one particular size will depend upon a number of elements such as the "size of the suspected abnormality" (Kirkpatrick et al., 1978), radiation dose to the patient, and so on.

The image contrast can be enhanced by the use of appropriate window width and window level settings (see Chapter 5). Once the picture is obtained, the radiologist may vary these settings on the console to suit his particular needs; that is, he can manipulate these settings until the optimal picture contrast is obtained for the particular structure (e.g., lesion) in which he is interested. For example, Kirkpatrick et al. (1978) have shown that by altering the window width and window level settings, other structures became more readily apparent.

Text continued on page 178

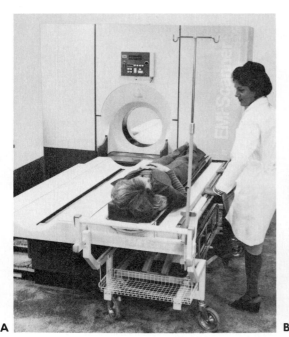

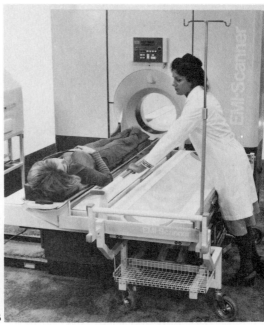

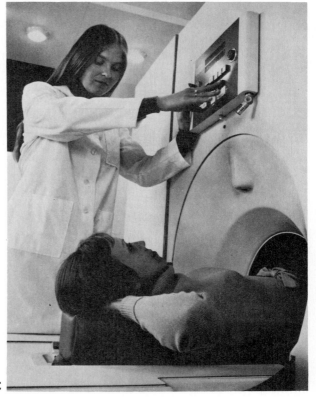

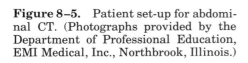

Figure 8–5. Patient set-up for abdominal CT. (Photographs provided by the Department of Professional Education, EMI Medical, Inc., Northbrook, Illinois.)

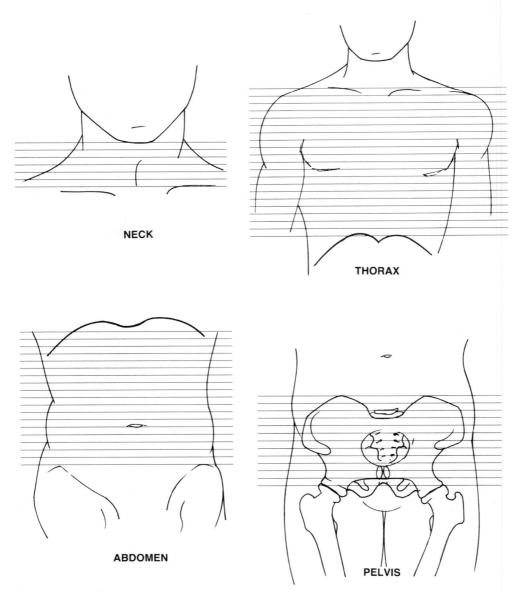

Figure 8–6. Typical scan sequences for the neck, thorax, abdomen, and pelvis. In the abdomen, for example, the sequence includes scanning from the base of the diaphragm to the iliac crest.

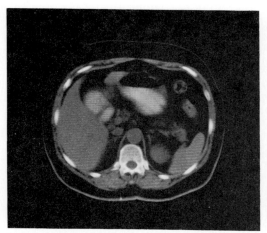

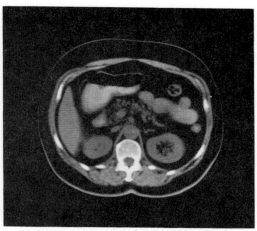

A, CT scan of the abdomen. Both adrenal glands are well visualized. The portal vein can be seen anterior to the inferior vena cava.

B, CT scan of the abdomen. The inferior portion of the left adrenal gland is well visualized, as is the vertical portion of the superior mesenteric artery anterior to the aorta.

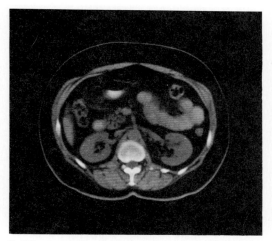

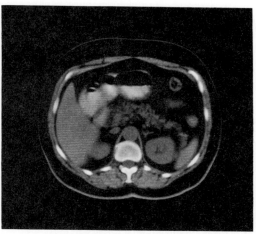

C, CT scan of the abdomen. The superior mesenteric artery is well visualized. The left renal vein can be seen crossing the abdomen and entering the inferior vena cava.

D, CT scan of the abdomen. Left adrenal gland is beautifully demonstrated. A portion of the right adrenal gland can be seen just posterior to the inferior vena cava.

Figure 8–7. Abdominal CT images demonstrating some anatomical areas of interest. (Courtesy of Pfizer/American Science and Engineering.)

Illustration continued on following page

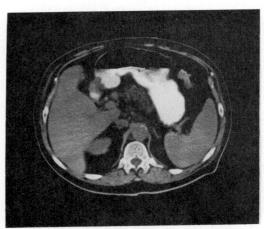

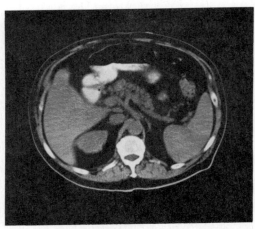

E, CT scan of the abdomen. There is contrast media in the stomach and small bowel. The body of the pancreas and the left adrenal gland are well visualized.

F, CT scan of the abdomen. The celiac artery can be seen branching into the hepatic and splenic arteries. The body of the pancreas, the splenic vein, and the left adrenal gland are well visualized.

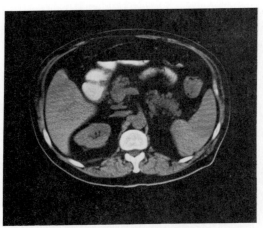

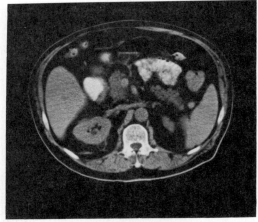

G, CT scan of the abdomen. The superior mesenteric artery, the body of the pancreas, the inferior vena cava, and the right kidney are beautifully demonstrated.

H, CT scan of the abdomen. The tail of the pancreas, the renal vein, and the right kidney are well visualized.

Figure 8–7*E,F,G,H   Continued*

Illustration continued on opposite page

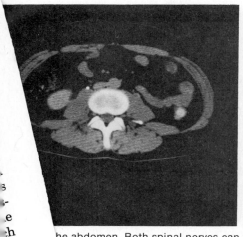

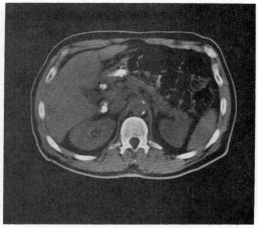

he abdomen. Both spinal nerves can
y exit from the neural foramina.

J, CT scan of the abdomen. The left adrenal gland
and tail and body of the pancreas are well visualized.

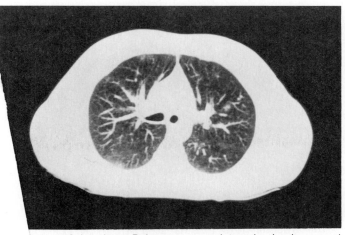

scan of the chest. Pulmonary vasculature is clearly seen at
riphery of the lungs.

Figure 8–7*I,J,K   Continued*

s
-
e
h

er
en-

y of

ay
is
By
be

79) for

These

racy
sults
ancy;
false-
itable
nd the
y, it is
ion or

CT OF THE BREAST

Investigation of the breast by CT is somewhat limited.

EQUIPMENT

For several years, two research prototype CT machines for mammography (CT/M) have undergone clinical testing at the Mayo Clinic and the University of Kansas Medical Center. (The unit at the Mayo Clinic has been discontinued.)

The CT/M unit made by General Electric uses a continuously rotating pulsed fan-beam (26°) of radiation, a water box, and an array of xenon detectors. The x-ray generator can operate between a variable range of kV and mA settings, but usually a setting of 116 kVp and 30 mA is used. The absorption values for the breast range from -127 to $+127$, with water being (Gisvold et al., 1977).

The patient is placed in the prone position, and the breast is inserted into hole in the tabletop. The top is then moved back to a horizontal position, shown in Figure 8-8, and the breast is lowered into the water box. Transmission readings are recorded and reconstruction techniques are applied to data. The reconstructed image is displayed on a 128×128 matrix in which each pixel is 1.5×1.5 mm. (Gisvold et al., 1977).

Radiation dose studies indicate that the levels (about 250 mR) are lower than in conventional mammography; however, spatial resolution in conventional mammography is higher than in CT of the breast.

SOME CLINICAL FINDINGS

Recent clinical results of Chang et al. (1979) from the University Kansas Medical Center suggest that:

CT/M studies of the breast yield specific information about lesions and provide the diagnosis when mammography fails to demonstrate the lesion unable to display the information necessary to make a definitive diagnosis using contrast medium to increase attenuation, very small carcinomas may identified, even in dysplastic breasts.

The interested student should refer to the work of Chang et al. (1979) details relating to the number of patients scanned and methodology.

Another recent work in this area is one by Gisvold et al. (1979) investigators have summarized their findings as follows:

...CT/M with infusion of contrast material (1) had a high degree of accuracy regarding malignant lesions, but not significantly better than the achieved with mammography; (2) was able to reveal clinically occult malignancy (3) was able to reveal mammographically occult malignancy; (4) gave positive results with a variety of benign lesions; and (5) is not considered suitable for routine screening of asymptomatic women, especially because of cost risk of contrast material infusion. If it has a place in medical practice today in the further evaluation of problematic cases found by physical examination mammography.

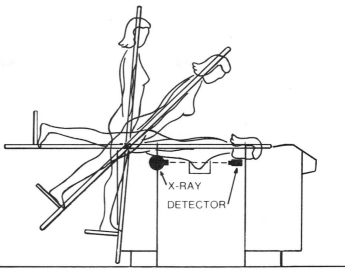

Figure 8-8. Patient positioning steps for CT of the breast. The breast is enclosed in a water bath. (From Edelheit, L. S., Herman, G. T., and Lakshminarayanan, A. V.: Reconstruction of objects from diverging x-rays. Med. Phys., 4:230, 1977. Reproduced by permission.)

OTHER TECHNIQUES

MULTIPLANAR RECONSTRUCTION

Apart from imaging cross-sectional anatomy, it is now possible to obtain CT scans in the *sagittal* and *coronal* planes (Fig. 8–9) (Haverling and Johanson, 1978; Maso et al., 1978).

In the past, sagittal and coronal CT images of the head were acquired by simply repositioning the patient's head. Anderson and Koehler (1979) have described patient positioning for coronal and sagittal CT scanning. In coronal scanning, for example, the patient's neck may be either flexed or extended to achieve satisfactory coronal images.

More recently, computer programs have been developed to generate these images using the information obtained from the standard transverse CT scans, thus obviating the need to reposition the patient.

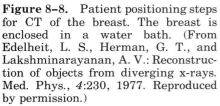

SAGITTAL PLANE

CORONAL PLANE

Figure 8–9. Diagrammatic representation of sagittal and coronal planes of the head.

Coronal and sagittal CT images provide a number of advantages, since they can (a) assist in accurate localization of structures, hence providing anatomical reference in surgery; (b) assist tremendously in radiation treatment planning by providing "a graphic display of the volume and extent of tumor masses. . ." (Federle et al., 1979); and (c) assist in evaluation of trauma. However, there are several disadvantages to multiplanar reconstruction, and these relate to the production of artifacts, higher dose, and difficulties in patient positioning for those scanners that do not have special computer programs for multiplanar reconstruction.

COMPUTED RADIOGRAPHIC LOCALIZATION IMAGES

Computed radiographic localization is a relatively new technique in clinical CT. Other commercial terms have been used to describe the same process, including (a) scout view (GE), (b) topogram (Siemens), and (c) pilot scan (Picker).

In computed radiographic localization, the x-ray tube and detectors remain stationary while the patient moves through the gantry aperture, as shown in Figure 8–10. The tube is then energized to produce x-rays in rapid pulses, which are sent to the computer for synthesis. The result is an image that looks similar to the conventional radiographic image. Several of these images are shown in Figure 8–11.

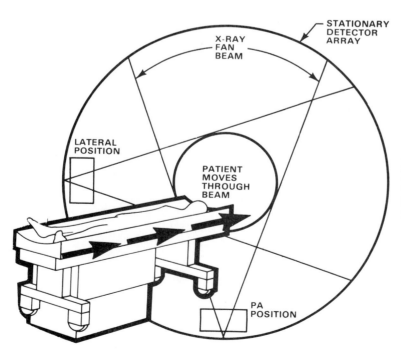

Figure 8–10. Simple illustration of the technique of computed radiography. (Courtesy of Picker International.)

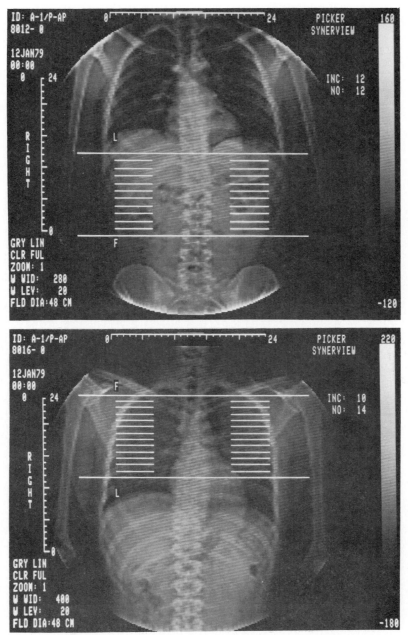

Figure 8–11. Four computed radiographic images indicating regions to be scanned. (Courtesy of Picker International.)

Illustration continued on following page

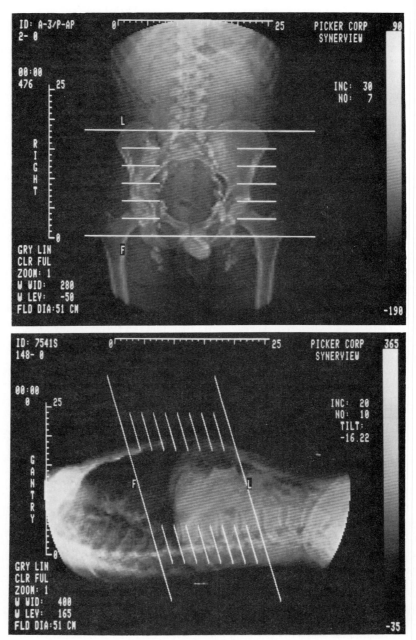

Figure 8–11   *Continued*

SUMMARY/REFERENCES/BIBLIOGRAPHY/REVIEW QUESTIONS

Summary

1. Several elements relating to the clinically oriented aspects of CT scanning include indications and efficacy, patient preparation and positioning, technical factors, and the use of contrast agents.

2. The clinical efficacy of CT of the head and body is well established. CT scanning of the head and body has received widespread acceptance, since it is primarily noninvasive and produces diagnostic information with great speed and accuracy.

3. Patient positioning of the head in CT involves the use of Reid's base line in determining various degrees of angulation. Usually scans are done at 0°, 20 to 25°, and 35° to Reid's base line. The degree of angulation depends on the structures to be examined.

4. Scanning the head involves taking a number of slices, commencing at the base and terminating at the vertex.

5. The use of contrast media in brain scanning has been proven to be efficacious in improving visualization of certain structures, especially intravascular blood and discrimination of neoplastic from non-neoplastic lesions.

6. The method of contrast administration can be either by bolus or by infusion.

7. Indications for body CT are numerous and are listed in the Appendix.

8. Patient preparation for body CT is important, since poor preparation will result in image degradation.

9. Good bowel preparation is essential for CT of the abdomen.

10. Antiperistaltic agents, contrast media (administered intravenously, orally, or through the rectum), preliminary scout views, selection of appropriate technical factors such as exposure factors, collimator width, window width, and window level settings are discussed.

11. In body scanning, the patient usually assumes a supine position, although prone and decubitus positioning is not uncommon.

12. Some clinical findings of CT of the breast were quoted from two studies, and other techniques in clinical CT were discussed briefly. These include multiplanar reconstruction and preliminary views.

13. In multiplanar reconstruction, it is possible to obtain coronal and sagittal CT sections of the body part either by repositioning the patient or by using special computer programs. Advantages and disadvantages of multiplanar reconstruction were pointed out.

14. Computed radiographic localization in CT is a relatively new technique in which an image similar to the conventional radiographic image can be generated.

References

Alfidi, R. J. (Ed.): Whole Body Computed Tomography. Radiol. Clin. North Am., Vol. XV, No. 3, Dec., 1977.

Anderson, R. E., and Koehler, P. R.: An accessory patient table for multidirectional CT scanning. Radiology, *130*:802–803, 1979.

Bories, J. (Ed.): The Diagnostic Limitations of Computerized Axial Tomography. New York, Springer-Verlag, 1978.

Carter, B. L., and Ignatow, S. G.: Computed body tomography. How useful is it? Postgrad. Med., *63*:66–80, 1978.

Chang, C. H., et al.: Specific value of computed tomographic breast scanner (CT/M) in diagnosis of breast diseases. Radiology, *132*:647–652, 1979.

Churchill, R. J., Reynes, C. J., Love, L., and Moncada, R.: CT imaging of the abdomen. *In* Love, L. (Ed.): Abdominal Imaging. Methodology and normal anatomy. Radiol. Clin. North Am., Vol. XVII, No. 1, April, 1979, pp. 13–24.

Cohen, W. N., et al.: Use of a tampon to enhance vaginal localization in computed tomography. Am. J. Roentgenol., *128*:1064–1065, 1977.

Federle, M. P., et al.: Coronal and sagittal reconstructions using a 4.8-second CT body scanner. Developments and applications. Am. J. Roentgenol., *133*:625–632, 1979.

Felson, B. (Ed.): Computerized Cranial Tomography. New York, Grune and Stratton, Inc., 1977.

Gado, M. H.: Contrast enhancement. *In* Proceedings of the Conference on Computerized Tomography in Radiology. St. Louis, American College of Radiology, 1976.

Gisvold, J. J., Karsell, P. R., and Reese, D. F.: Computerized tomographic mammography. *In* Logan, W. W. (Ed.): Breast Carcinoma. New York, John Wiley, Inc., 1977.

Gisvold, J. J., Reese, D. F., and Karsell, P. R.: Computed tomographic mammography (CTM). Am. J. Roentgenol., *133*:1143–1149, 1979.

Hanaway, J., Scott, W. R., and Strother, C. M.: An Atlas of the Human Brain and the Orbit for Computed Tomography. St. Louis, Warren Green, Inc., 1977.

Haverling, M., and Johanson, H.: Computed sagittal tomography of the orbit. Am. J. Roentgenol., *131*:346–347, 1978.

Huckman, M. S.: Clinical experience with the intravenous infusion of iodinated contrast material as an adjunct to computed tomography. Surg. Neurol., *4*:297–318, 1975.

Huckman, M. S., Grainer, L. S., and Classen, R. C.: The normal computed tomogram. *In* Felson, B. (Ed.): Computerized Cranial Tomography. New York, Grune and Stratton, Inc., 1977.

Kirkpatrick, R. H., et al.: Scanning techniques in computed body tomography. Am. J. Roentgenol., *130*:1069–1075, 1978.

Kramer, R. A., et al.: An approach to contrast enhancement in computed tomography of the brain. Radiology, *16*:641–647, 1975.

Lampert, V. L., Zelch, J. V., and Cohen, D. N.: Computed tomography of the orbits. Radiology, *113*:351–354, 1974.

Ledley, R. S.: Editorial. Computerized tomography. International Journal of Radiological Diagnosis Using CT Scanners, Vol. 1, No. 1. New York, Pergamon Press, 1977.

Lin, J. P.: Computed tomography of the head in adults. Postgrad. Med., *60*:113–119, 1976.

Lin, J. P., et al.: Brain tumors studied by computerized tomography. *In* Thompson, R. A., and Green, J. R. (Eds.): Neoplasia in the Central Nervous System. New York, Raven Press, 1976.

Love, L. (Ed.): Abdominal Imaging. Radiol. Clin. North Am., Vol. XVII, No. 1, April, 1979.

Manfredi, O. L.: Cost-effectiveness of CT and ultrasound. Appl. Radiol., 73–76, March/April, 1979.

Maso, S., Norman, D., and Newton, T. H.: Coronal computed tomography: Indications and accuracy. Am. J. Roentgenol., *131*:875–879, 1978.

Meschan, I.: Synopsis of Radiologic Anatomy with Computed Tomography. Philadelphia, W. B. Saunders Company, 1978.

Naidich, T. P., and Kricheff, I. I.: Computed tomography of the head in children. Postgrad. Med., *60*:123–129, 1976.

New, P. F. J.: Computed tomography: A major diagnostic advance. Hosp. Pract., *10*:55–64, 1975.

Norman, D., et al. (Eds.): Computed Tomography 1977. St. Louis, The C. V. Mosby Co., 1977.

Norman, D., Enzman, D. R., and Newton, T. H.: Optimal contrast dosage in cranial computed tomography. Am. J. Roentgenol., *131*:687–689, 1978.

Ruijs, S. H. J.: A simple procedure for patient preparation in abdominal CT. Am. J. Roentgenol., *133*:551–552, 1979.

Seidelman, F. E., et al.: Computed tomography of the gas-filled bladder — Method of staging bladder neoplasms. Urology, *9*:337–344, 1977.

Skalnik, B.: CT body scanning — A question of efficacy. Appl. Radiol., 91–95, July/Aug., 1977.

Sodee, D. B. (Ed.): Correlations in Diagnostic Imaging. New York, Appleton-Century-Crofts, 1979.

Stephens, D. H., Sheedy, P. F., II, et al.: Initial clinical experience with computed tomography of the body. Radiol. Clin. North Am., *14*:149–158, 1976.

Bibliography

Carter, B. L., and Ignatow, S. G.: Computed body tomography. How useful is it? Postgrad. Med.,
   63:66–80, 1978.
Kirkpatrick, R. H., et al.: Scanning techniques in computed body tomography. Am. J. Roentgenol.,
   130:1069–1075, 1978.
Kramer, R. A., et al.: An approach to contrast enhancement in computed tomography of the brain.
   Radiology, *16*:641–647, 1975.
Lin, J. P.: Computed tomography of the head in adults. Postgrad. Med., *60*:113–119, 1976.
Naidich, T. P., and Kricheff, I. I.: Computed tomography of the head in children. Postgrad. Med.,
   60:123–129, 1976.
Ruijs, S. H. J.: A simple procedure for patient preparation in abdominal CT. Am. J. Roentgenol.,
   133:551–552, 1979.
Skalnik, B.: CT body scanning — A question of efficacy. Appl. Radiol., 91–95, July/Aug., 1977.

Review Questions

1. CT may be used in the study of:
   (a) Cerebral infarction.
   (b) Intraorbital lesions.
   (c) Posterior fossa tumors.
   (d) All of the above.

2. Artifacts that have a streak-like appearance on the CT image of the head may
be produced by:
   (a) Hairpins.
   (b) Breathing.
   (c) Air in the ventricles.
   (d) Radiolucent tape around patient's head.

3. A typical angulation range for demonstration of posterior fossa structures in
CT scanning of the head is:
   (a) 0° to 10°
   (b) 25° to 35°
   (c) 20° to 25°
   (d) 30° to 35°

4. Which of the following is used as a reference base line for positioning of the
head in CT scanning?
   (a) Radiographic base line.
   (b) Mid-sagittal plane.
   (c) A line drawn from the supraorbital margin to the external auditory
       meatus.
   (d) A line drawn from the infraorbital margin to the external auditory
       meatus.

5. Which of the following is an established and useful technique in CT scanning?
   (a) Intravenous administration of contrast media.
   (b) Oral administration of contrast media.
   (c) Administration of contrast via the rectum.
   (d) All of the above.

6. The use of intravenous contrast in CT will result in:
   (a) Increased allergic reactions.
   (b) Contrast enhancement of internal structures.
   (c) The use of longer scan times and higher kVp.
   (d) A blood-iodine level of 100 mg./100 ml. of contrast.

7. Carcinomas of the breast may be detected by CT because:
    (a) Contrast media are used to increase attenuation.
    (b) A special matrix is used.
    (c) The machine is superior to conventional radiographic equipment.
    (d) A special detection system is used.

8. Which of the following is referring to computed radiography?
    (a) Use of the computer to determine appropriate exposure factors.
    (b) Use of the computer to move the patient through the gantry aperture in 1-cm. increments.
    (c) Use of the computer to produce a cross-sectional image in three dimensions.
    (d) Use of the computer to produce an image that looks similar to the conventional x-ray image.

9. In CT scanning of the head, a number of scans taken parallel to Reid's base line are useful primarily in examining:
    (a) Posterior fossa structures.
    (b) Orbits, sella turcica, and suprasellar areas.
    (c) Facial bones.
    (d) Soft tissues.

10. In CT scanning of the head, it is customary to scan:
    (a) From base to vertex.
    (b) From vertex to base.
    (c) From vertex to midbrain only.
    (d) From midbrain to base only.

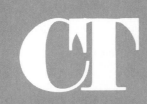

CHAPTER 9

OTHER DEVELOPMENTS IN CT

A multiple x-ray source, high speed, transaxial scanner system (DSR) is about to undergo evaluation studies. The capability for programmable scanning modes and operative-interactive retrospective reconfiguration of scan data makes the DSR a very powerful research tool.

ERIK L. RITMAN, JAMES H. KINSEY, RICHARD A. ROBB,
LOWELL D. HARRIS, BARRY K. GILBERT (1980)

DEVELOPMENTS IN CT

The topics to be discussed in this section are relatively new techniques. Some of them have been under clinical evaluation, while others have undergone experimental tests. Because of this, only a short review will be given, since only time and results of research will indicate their universal use in radiology.

CT IN CARDIAC APPLICATIONS

A categorization of CT scanners (Table 9–1) for cardiac applications (Tables 9–2 and 9–3) has been given by Brody (1978). These imaging methods will now be briefly described.

Some workers (e.g., Lipton et al., 1978; Miller et al., 1977) have reported demonstrating several useful results of cardiac CT using contrast media and

TABLE 9–1. CATEGORIZATION OF CT SCANNERS FOR CARDIAC APPLICATIONS

MODE	BRIEF EXPLANATION
Static	Single scans with an effective scan time of 1 to 5 sec.
Dynamic	Multiple 1- to 5-sec. scans taken in rapid succession.
Gated	Synchronous reconstruction of the heart with an effective scan time less than 500 msec. through gating the scan views to the electrocardiogram (ECG).
Rapid	Scanners with static scan intervals of less than 500 msec.

From Brody, W.: Current status of cardiovascular imaging by transmission computed tomography. *In* Miller, H.A., Schmidt, E.V., and Harrison, D.C. (Eds.): Noninvasive Cardiovascular Measurements. Washington, D.C., Society of Photo Optical Instrumentation Engineers, 1978. Used by permission.

CT scanners that have shorter than 5-second scan times. However, this mode of cardiac CT poses several limitations due to motion of organs and breathing, which degrade image resolution, the ability of the scanner to scan only one cross section, and timing between the x-ray exposure and injection of contrast material (Brody, 1978).

CT can also be used to provide information on the dynamics of organ systems by taking a series of scans with each separated only slightly in time, that is, in rapid sequence using contrast media (bolus injection). This is *dynamic CT* imaging, which can be achieved by either of two methods. In one method (Berninger et al., 1978; Hacker and Becker, 1977), the gantry of the CT unit rotates in a clockwise and then in a counterclockwise direction for rapid back-to-back CT scans with a time interval between scans of about 4 seconds. In the other method, the gantry (of a fan-beam scanner) rotates continuously by making use of a specially designed apparatus (slip-ring connector) to enable acquisition of images in rapid sequence (Brody, 1978).

This kind of cardiac CT imaging has brought forth some fruitful results. "The sequential opacification of cardiac chambers, easily demonstrable with dynamic CT, represents a significant improvement in cardiac chamber visualization over static CT" (Brody, 1978).

The limitations imposed by dynamic CT (high patient dose, problems in image quality due to noise, etc.) generate the notion of the need for other systems that will provide the resolution for cardiac applications.

Gated CT techniques have been described by Sagel et al. (1977), Harell et

TABLE 9–2. CURRENT AND FUTURE APPLICATIONS OF CARDIOVASCULAR COMPUTED TOMOGRAPHY

CURRENT USES	FUTURE APPLICATIONS
Aortic aneurysms	Aortic dissections
LV aneurysms	LV, RV contractility
Cardiac chamber size	Myocardial mass
Great vessel orientation	Evaluation of congenital heart disease
Cardiac and vascular calcification	
Pericardial effusion	Coronary artery imaging
Coronary bypass graft patency	Myocardial ischemia
Myocardial infarction	Regional pulmonary perfusion

From Brody, W.: Current status of cardiovascular imaging by transmission computed tomography. *In* Miller, H.A., Schmidt, E.V., and Harrison, D.C. (Eds.): Noninvasive Cardiovascular Measurements. Washington, D.C., Society of Photo Optical Instrumentation Engineers, 1978. Used by permission.

TABLE 9–3. POTENTIAL APPLICATIONS OF CARDIOVASCULAR COMPUTED TOMOGRAPHY

DIAGNOSTIC FUNCTION	ANATOMIC STRUCTURE	INFORMATION DESIRED
Definition of Cardiac Anatomy		
Structure	Chambers	
	Valves	Location, size, connections, calcifications
	Great vessels	
Function	Ventricles	Cardiac output
		Ejection fraction
		Segmental wall motion
Assessment of Blood Flow/Perfusion		
	Blood vessels	
	Bypass grafts	Patency, stenosis
	Great vessels	Thromboembolism, aneurysms
	Coronary arteries	Atherosclerotic narrowing
	Myocardium	Ischemia
		Infarction

From Brody, W.: Current status of cardiovascular imaging by transmission computed tomography. *In* Miller, H.A., Schmidt, E.V., and Harrison, D.C. (Eds.): Noninvasive Cardiovascular Measurements. Washington, D.C., Society of Photo Optical Instrumentation Engineers, 1978. Used by permission.

al. (1977), and Ter-Pogossian et al. (1976). In its most fundamental description, gated CT refers to the use of the information from an electrocardiogram (ECG) in conjunction with a CT scanner, so that the heartbeat and the scanner are synchronized (Brody, 1978). The term *gated* is used to denote a special apparatus that puts out data in response to specific input data (e.g., from the ECG).

Finally, Robb and Ritman (1979) have pointed out that

... gated CT scanning based on the electrocardiogram cannot be used for stop action synchronous volume imaging of the myocardium or for angiographic imaging of vascular anatomy or circulatory function. This is because the beat-to-beat myocardial geometry and the transient dynamic distribution pattern and concentration of contrast material during and following its injection vary continuously and non-reproducibly. Moreover the pharmacologic effect of contrast material alters the hemodynamic and cardiodynamic status considerably so that beat-to-beat constancy of the heartbeat cannot be achieved during or for a considerable period after the injection of contrast material particularly into the coronary arteries.

The technique of *rapid CT* imaging can solve the problems imposed by gated CT imaging. Recently, a number of techniques for rapid CT have been proposed (Quinn et al., 1978; Iinuma et al., 1977). One such system is the *dynamic spatial reconstructor* (DSR) (Ritman et al., 1980). The DSR provides high temporal resolution, a parameter that present-day CT scanners cannot provide (Wood et al., 1979). The term *temporal resolution* is used to refer to two parameters, those of "shutter speed or the effective exposure time required to scan the object and the frame rate, the number of scans per minute" (Brody, 1978).

THE DYNAMIC SPATIAL RECONSTRUCTOR

The DSR is a sophisticated computerized tomographic machine capable of evaluating structural anatomy, dynamics of organ systems, and functional

189

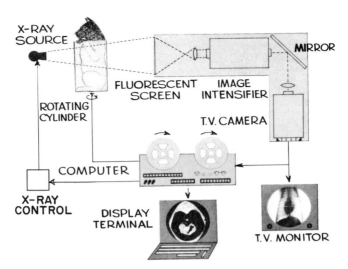

Figure 9–1. Diagrammatic representation of the principles of the single source dynamic spatial reconstructor (SSDSR) used at the Mayo Clinic. The x-ray tube is directly under the control of the computer to pulse x-rays at 0.34 sec. in synchrony with computer-controlled stepwise rotation of the dog and the heartbeat. The purpose of the image intensifier is to brighten the fluoroscopic image that is displayed on the television monitor. The video signal from the television camera can also be used to provide information on the intensities of the transmitted x-rays. This is accomplished by the computer, which performs reconstruction to generate cross-sectional images (up to 240) for any projection angle. (From Robb, R. A., and Ritman, E. L.: High speed synchronous volume computed tomography of the heart. Radiology, *133*:655–661, 1979. Reproduced by permission.)

details of the cardiovascular and pulmonary systems (Wood et al., 1977). This machine has been under investigation and development through a collaborative effort by a research group at the Mayo Clinic and the Raytheon Company for the past few years.

The principles of the DSR are based on the single source (one x-ray tube) dynamic spatial reconstructor (SSDR) (Fig. 9–1) currently used at the Mayo Clinic. In Figure 9–2, a diagrammatic representation of the DSR is shown. It consists of 28 rotating-anode x-ray tubes coupled to 28 *image intensifier*

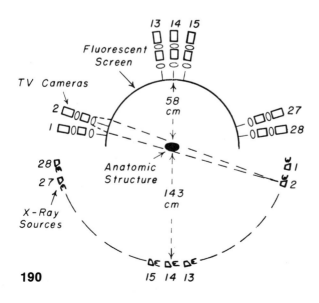

Figure 9–2. Schematic arrangement of patient, x-ray tubes, and detectors in the DSR system. The patient remains stationary while the x-ray tubes and detectors (image intensifiers/video chain) move simultaneously around the patient. (From Wood, E. H.: New horizons for study of the cardiopulmonary and circulatory systems. Chest, *69*:394–408, 1976. Reproduced by permission.)

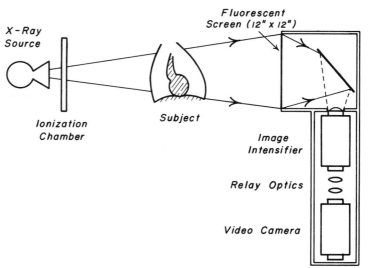

Figure 9–3. Schematic of a single imaging chain (see text) of the DSR system. The ionization chamber is used to measure the intensity of the radiation. Other details of the chain include the light-to-light image intensifier tubes and the isocon TV camera tube because of several advantages relating to its (isocon tube) resolution sensitivity and dynamic range. (From Wood, E. H.: New horizons for study of the cardiopulmonary and circulatory systems. Chest, *69*: 394–408, 1976. Reproduced by permission.)

screens, each with its own television chain. The x-ray tubes (below patient) and the intensifiers both form a semicircular array about the patient, and both are housed in a rotating gantry.

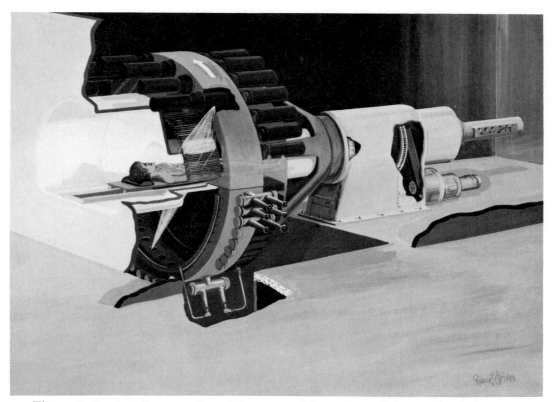

Figure 9–4. Artist's conception of the proposed dynamic spatial reconstructor. (From Wood, E. H., Robb, R. A., and Ritman, E. L.: Possible role of computed tomography in the non-invasive diagnosis of heart disease. *In* Kaltenbach, M., Lichtben, P., Balcon, R., and Bussman, W. D.: Coronary heart disease. Stuttgart, Georg Thieme, 1978, pp. 106–115. Reproduced by permission.)

A schematic representation of one of the imaging chains, which include the x-ray tube, fluorescent screen, and television chain, is shown in Figure 9–3. In Figure 9–4 an artist's conception of the DSR is shown.

The scanning sequence and data collection are based on the following:

1. The gantry rotates continuously at 50 rpm through 360° by computer control to scan about cylindrical volumes in the patient.

2. The x-ray tubes are pulsed during rotation.

3. Each scan will generate data to reconstruct about 250 cross-sectional images.

4. The multiplanar video signals are recorded by video disks or tapes and are sent to the computer for processing and data analysis.

The DSR produces a true three-dimensional image of the structure examined. Two such images are shown in the top half of Figure 9–5, while the bottom half shows an image that demonstrates the ability of the DSR to "cut open" the structure. Such an image is made possible only by the use of rigorous mathematical techniques. A further description of the physical and technological aspects of the DSR is given in a recent paper by Ritman et al. (1980).

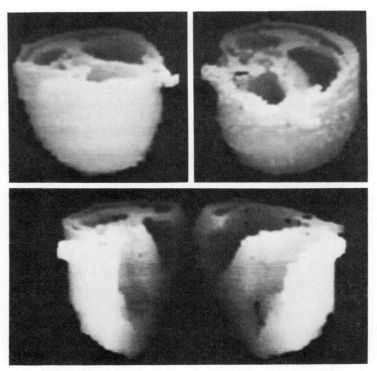

Figure 9–5. This image of an intact dog's heart shows the three-dimensional imaging capability expected of the Mayo Clinic's Dynamic Spatial Reconstructor (DSR). A computer program detects the heart muscle, both inner and outer surfaces, and generates a perspective "three-dimensional" picture such as illustrated here. Slicing the heart open with a "mathematical scalpel" will enable investigators to look into interior chambers. The computer program used to generate this image was developed by Dr. H. K. Liu in partial fulfillment of his Ph.D. thesis. (Picture reproduced with permission from Robb, R. A., Harris, L. D., and Ritman, E. L.: Computerized x-ray reconstruction tomography in stereometric analysis of cardiovascular dynamics. Proceedings of the Society of Photo Optical Instrumentation Engineers, 1976.)

It is possible that within the next decade, a modified DSR may become available for space flight studies in the National Aeronautics and Space Administration (NASA) space shuttle vehicles (Wood, 1978).

OTHER FUTURE TRENDS

A thorough discussion of future trends is not possible in a text of this kind, since changes in the technology are occurring at a rapid rate. However, a few points are noteworthy. Other future trends indicate work related to the following:

1. Higher spatial resolution through reduction of aperture size and reconstruction of part of the CT image on smaller pixels (General Electric Company, 1979a; Blumenfeld, 1981).

2. Improvement of CT number accuracy and reduction of artifacts (General Electric Company, 1979a; Blumenfeld, 1981).

3. Studies on the use of different semiconductors in CT imaging and other work pertaining to detectors (e.g., photodiodes with integrated pre-amplifiers) (General Electric Company, 1979a).

4. The growth of quality assurance programs and performance evaluation.

5. The growth of CT in radiation therapy applications.

6. A host of other research projects relating to computing, mathematics, image quality, radiation dose, physics and engineering aspects, planning, economics, and clinical applications.

7. Changes in x-ray sources and the use of shorter scan times (Buchmann, 1981).

USE OF CT IN RADIATION TREATMENT PLANNING

Several investigators (Chernak et al., 1975; Smith et al., 1976; Geise and McCullough, 1977; Manzenrider et al., 1977; Prasad et al., 1979) have applied CT to radiation treatment planning (RTP).

One system for RTP is shown in Figure 9–6. The area of the patient to be

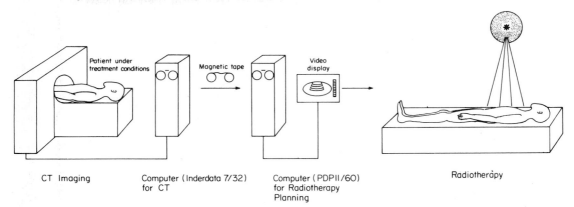

Figure 9–6. A radiotherapy treatment planning system using computed tomography. (From Battista et al.: The application of computed tomography (CT) imaging to radiotherapy planning. Proceedings of Society of Photo Optical Instrumentation Engineers. Vol. 173: Application of Optical Instrumentation in Medicine VII. Washington, D.C., 1979. Reproduced by permission.)

STEP 1
CT image with regions of interest identified using cursor.

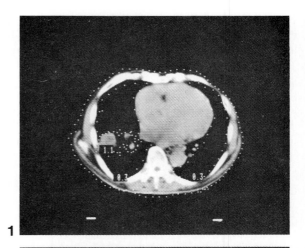

1

STEP 2
Program beam locations and computation area of interest.

TREATMENT
BEAM 2

ISODOSE
CONTOUR
COMPUTATION
AREA

TREATMENT
BEAM 1

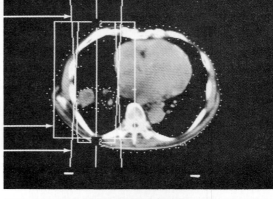

2

STEP 3
Observe computed isodose profiles and determine appropriate Treatment Plan.

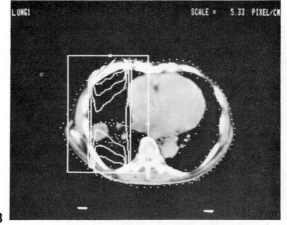

3

Figure 9–7.   Images showing typical steps in the application of CT to radiotherapy treatment planning with a Synerview CT system. (Courtesy of Picker International.)

treated by radiotherapy is first examined by CT. The information from the CT scan goes to the computer in radiotherapy for planning of beam positions, calculation of depth doses, and calculation and display of isodose curves, which can be superimposed on the CT image.

In essence, the CT numbers are used in calculating physical and electron densities, which are then used in dose computations. Radiotherapy is finally applied to the patient in the exact position used in CT (Battista et al., 1979).

The steps in the process are illustrated in Figure 9–7.

SOME ECONOMIC CONSIDERATIONS

CT AND HEALTH CARE

There is a great deal of concern among national health care planners, the health insurance industry, and health care administrators about the high cost of CT technology. This has led to a controversy related to the economics of CT, particularly how it affects health care costs.

In view of this, the United States Department of Health and Human Services issued planning guidelines that were intended to limit the availability of the CT scanner by restricting the purchase of these units to those hospitals expected to carry out at least 2500 procedures per year, since the United States Office of Technology Assessment showed that about 2700 procedures per year can be done by an average scanner.

CT manufacturers opposed these guidelines and argued that these (the guidelines) would impede further development and spread of CT machines. Hence, the CT scanner became a controversial topic. It also became an important economic issue because of increasing medical care costs, which were partially attributed to the scanner and to large capital investments and other factors that will be discussed.

Despite these concerns, the technology continued to elicit enthusiasm, and a number of studies were launched to investigate some economic aspects of CT. Such studies include the works of Evans and Jost (1976, 1979), Wortzman and Holgate (1979), Thomson (1977), Abrams and McNeil (1978), Bartlett et al. (1978), Manfredi (1979), and Freedman (1978), to mention only a few.

SOME COST ASPECTS

Most of the actual figures reported in the literature will not be quoted here, since costs and charges will change significantly with time. The reader should refer to the original source for such figures.

Several aspects relating to the cost of CT facilities which should be considered initially are (Bartlett et al., 1978):

1. Purchase and installation costs

2. Consumables (including costs of magnetic tapes, disks, contrast media, film, and so on)

3. Maintenance costs

4. Staffing costs

5. Equipment update costs

Purchase costs, for example, are high, with capital investments of $350,000 to $950,000 and operating costs of $250,000 to $400,000 per year (Abrams and McNeil, 1978).

Another issue regarding the CT cost controversy deals with benefit implications. Are the benefits weighed against the cost of the technology? The answer to this question lies in the use of two assessment methods: (a) cost-effectiveness and (b) cost-benefit.

A *cost-effectiveness analysis* involves the choice of a specific goal and a comparison of CT to other ways by which to achieve the same goal (Brown, 1970). In CT, for example, such goals would be a cross-sectional image, the ability of the system to image very small differences in tissue density, and the noninvasive nature of the procedure.

The concept of a *cost-benefit analysis* involves the use of a *cost-benefit ratio*, which is a "ratio of the value of the benefit of an alternative to the value of the alternative's costs" (Manfredi, 1979). The cost of the alternative is acceptable if this ratio is more than one (Manfredi, 1979).

Cost-effectiveness analysis has been reported (Klarman, 1974) to be more suitable for use in health care than cost-benefit analysis, since "social and intangible benefits are converted into dollar figures — for example, poor health into dollars lost from work missed — an obviously difficult and controversial task" (Banta et al., 1979).

Although CT facilities cost a great deal of money, several studies (e.g., Bartlett et al., 1978; Wortzman and Holgate, 1979) have indicated a number of benefits. These benefits include a reduction of patient hospitalization costs, since patients can be examined on an "outpatient" basis, and also a reduction and even elimination of some invasive procedures (angiography and pneumoencephalography) and hence savings in consumables such as contrast media and films.

Apart from these cost savings, other benefits are also apparent. These include the clinical efficacy of CT, which was discussed in Chapter 8.

Equally important here also is the cost of CT technology in the future. In considering this aspect, one may hope that with the decreasing cost of computer hardware and the rapid development of computer technology, perhaps the cost of CT equipment may eventually be reasonably affordable.

A CLOSING REMARK

CT represents a giant technological development in the history of medicine. The spread of CT technology has been rapid and has resulted in tremendous enthusiasm throughout the world. Such enthusiasm has generated a compendium of information relating to mathematics, physics, engineering, clinical applications, and the economics of CT within a relatively short time span. More importantly, the use of CT as a clinical tool in the detection and management of a large number of disease processes has been well established, and the literature on clinical applications continues to grow.

In view of this, CT will continue to have a profound effect on diagnostic imaging and will play an important role in health care. As research investigations continue, CT will become commonplace in the future.

The student must therefore make every effort now to understand the fundamental principles of CT in order to gain the full benefits of the technique.

CT / 9

REFERENCES/BIBLIOGRAPHY

References

Abrams, H. L., and McNeil, B. J.: Computed tomography: Cost and efficacy implications. Am. J. Roentgenol., *131*:81–87, 1978.

Banta, H. D., Corcoran, S., and Sanes, J. R.: Weighing the benefits and costs of medical technologies. Proceedings of the IEEE, *67*:1190–1195, 1979.

Bartlett, J. R., et al.: Evaluating cost-effectiveness of diagnostic equipment: the brain scanner case. Br. Med. J., *2*:815–820, 1978.

Battista, J. J., Van Dyk, J., et al.: The application of computed tomography (CT) imaging to radiotherapy planning. *In* Gray, J. (Ed.): Application of Optical Instrumentation in Medicine VII, Vol. 173. Washington, D.C., Society of Photo Optical Instrumentation Engineers, 1979.

Berninger, W. H., Redington, R. W., and Doherty, P.: Time resolution computed tomography. (Abstract) Med. Phys., *5*:336, 1978.

Blumenfeld, M.: CT — The future in focus. Australas. Radiol., *25*:181–197, 1981.

Brody, W.: Current status of cardio-vascular imaging by transmission computed tomography. *In* Miller, H. A., Schmidt, E. V., and Harrison, D. C. (Eds.): Noninvasive Cardiovascular Measurements. Washington, D.C., Society of Photo Optical Instrumentation Engineers, 1978.

Brown, M.: An economic analysis of hospital operations. Hosp. Adm., *15*:76–78, 1970.

Buchmann, F.: The future of computed tomography. Medicamundi, *26*:23–27, 1981.

Chernak, E. S., Rodriguez-Anturez, A., et al.: The use of computed tomography for radiation therapy treatment planning. Radiology, *117*:613–614, 1975.

Evans, R. G., and Jost, G.: Economic analysis of computed tomography units. Am. J. Roentgenol., *127*:191–198, 1976.

Evans, R. G., and Jost, G.: Utilization of body computed tomography units. Radiology, *131*:695–698, 1979.

Evans, R. G., and Jost, G.: Utilization of head computed tomography units. Radiology, *131*:691–693, 1979.

Freedman, G. S.: CT: A financial and legislative reappraisal. Appl. Radiol., 140–144, Nov.-Dec., 1978.

Geise, R. A., and McCullough, E. C.: The use of CT scanners in megavoltage photon-beam therapy planning. Radiology, *124*:133–141, 1977.

General Electric Company, Medical Systems Division: CT/T Continuum. Brochure No. 4928, 1979a.

General Electric Company, Medical Systems Division: CT/T Continuum: The Future in Focus. Brochure No. 4941, 1979b.

Gisvold, J. J., Karsell, P. R., and Reese, D. F.: Computerized tomographic mammography. *In* Logan, W. W. (Ed.): Breast Carcinoma. New York, John Wiley, Inc., 1977.

Hacker, H., and Becker, H.: Time controlled CT angiography. J. Comput. Assist. Tomog., *1*:405–410, 1977.

Harell, G. S., Guthaner, D. F., et al.: Stop action cardiac computed tomography. Radiology, *123*:515–517, 1977.

Iinuma, T. A., et al.: Proposed system for ultra fast computed tomography. J. Comput. Assist. Tomog., *1*:494–498, 1977.

Klarman, H. E.: Application of cost-benefit analysis to the health services and the special case of technologic innovation. Int. J. Health Serv., *4*:325–352, 1974.

Lipton, M. J., Hayashi, T. T., Boyd, D., and Carlsson, E.: Measurement of left ventricular cast volume by computed tomography. Radiology, *127*:419–423, 1978.

Manfredi, O. L.: Cost effectiveness of CT and ultrasound. Appl. Radiol., March-April, 1979.

Manzenrider, J. E., et al.: Use of body scanner in radiotherapy treatment planning. Cancer, *40*:170–179, 1977.

Miller, S. W., et al.: Right and left ventricular volumes and wall measurements. Determination by CT in arrested canine hearts. Am. J. Roentgenol., *129*:257–261, 1977.

Prasad, S. C., Glasgow, G. P., and Purdy, J. A.: Dosimetric evaluation of a computerized tomography treatment system. Radiology, *130*:777–781, 1979.

Quinn, J. R., et al.: A proposed practical high speed CT scanner for cardiac imaging. (Abstract) Med. Phys., *5*:531, 1978.

Raytheon Company: Personal Communications, 1979.

Ritman, E. L., Robb, R. A., et al.: Quantitative imaging of the structure and function of the heart, lungs and circulation. Mayo Clin. Proc., *53*:3–11, 1978.

Ritman, E. L., et al.: Physical and technical considerations in the design of the DSR: A high temporal resolution volume scanner. Am. J. Roentgenol., *134*:369–374, 1980.

Robb, R. A., and Ritman, E. L.: High speed synchronous volume computed tomography of the heart. Radiology, *133*:655–661, 1979.

Sagel, S. S., et al.: Gated computed tomography of the human heart. Invest. Radiol., *12*:563–566, 1977.

Smith, V., Boyd, D. P., et al.: A computerized transverse section transmission scanner for radiation therapy treatment planning. Presented at the Fourth International Conference on Medical Physics, Ottawa, Canada, July 25–30, 1976.

Ter-Pogossian, M. M., et al.: Computed tomography of the heart. Am. J. Roentgenol., *12*:79–90, 1976.

Thomson, J. L. G.: Cost-effectiveness of an EMI brain scanner. A review of a 2-year experience. Health Trends, *9*:16–19, 1977.

Wood, E. H.: New horizons for study of the cardiopulmonary and circulatory systems. Chest, *69*:394–408, 1976.

Wood, E. H., et al.: Non-invasive numerical vivisection of anatomic structure and function of the intact circulatory system using a high temporal resolution cylindrical scanning computerized tomograph. Med. Instrum., *11*:153–158, 1976.

Wood, E. H., et al.: Applications of high temporal resolution cylindrical scanning tomography to physiology and medicine. *In* Raviv, J., et al. (Eds.): Computer-Aided Tomography and Ultrasonics in Medicine. IFIP North-Hollands Publishing Company, 1979.

Wortzman, G., and Holgate, R. C.: Reappraisal of the cost-effectiveness of computed tomography in a government-sponsored health care system. Radiology, *130*:257–261, 1979.

Bibliography

Abrams, H. L., and McNeil, B. J.: Computed tomography: Cost and efficacy implications. Am. J. Roentgenol., *131*:81–87, 1978.

Chernak, E. S., Rodriguez-Anturez, A., et al.: The use of computed tomography for radiation therapy treatment planning. Radiology, *117*:513–614, 1975.

Evans, R. G., and Jost, G.: Economic analysis of computed tomographic units. Am. J. Roentgenol., *127*:191–198, 1976.

Ritman, E. L., et al.: Physical and technical considerations in the design of the DSR: A high temporal resolution volume scanner. Am. J. Roentgenol., *134*:369–374, 1980.

Wood, E. H.: New horizons for study of the cardiopulmonary and circulatory systems. Chest, *69*:394–408, 1976.

APPENDIX

INDICATIONS FOR BODY CT*

Neck

- Determination of the extent of primary and secondary neoplasms of the neck.
- Evaluation of bony abnormalities of the cervical spine including neoplasms, fractures, dislocations, and congenital anomalies.
- Localization of foreign bodies in the soft tissues, hypopharynx, or larynx and assessment of airway integrity after trauma.
- Evaluation of retropharyngeal abscesses.

Mediastinum

- Evaluation of problems presented by chest radiograph.
  - Mass.
    - Differentiation among cystic, fatty, or solid nature.
    - Localization relative to other mediastinal structures.
  - Mediastinal widening.
    - Assessment of whether cause is pathologic or anatomic variation.
    - Distinction of solid mass, vascular anomaly, or aneurysm, and physiologic fat deposition.
  - Hilum.
    - Differentiation of enlarged pulmonary artery from solid mass when conventional tomography fails or is not capable of making this distinction.
  - Paraspinal line widening.
    - Distinction among lymph node enlargement, vascular cause, or anatomic variant.
- Search for occult thymic lesion.
  - Detection of thymoma or hyperplasia in selected patients with myasthenia gravis when plain chest radiography is negative or suspicious.

Lung

- Search for pulmonary lesions.
  - Detection of occult pulmonary metastases when:
    - Extensive surgery is planned for a known primary neoplasm with a high propensity for lung metastases or for apparent solitary lung metastasis.
  - Detection of primary tumor in patient with positive sputum cytology and negative chest radiography and fiberoptic bronchoscopy.
  - Assessment of lung and mediastinum for underlying pleural effusion and the postpneumonectomy fibrothorax for recurrent disease.
- Search for diffuse or central calcification in a pulmonary nodule when conventional tomography is indeterminate.
- Determination of extent of intrathoracic spread in selected patients with bronchogenic carcinoma including mediastinal or pleural invasion.

Chest Wall

- Determination of extent of neoplastic disease.
  - Assess bone, muscle, and subcutaneous tissues.
  - Detection of intrusion into thoracic cavity or spinal canal.

Percutaneous Needle Biopsy

- Assist biopsy of lesions when fluoroscopic guidance inadequate.
  - Certain mediastinal masses.
  - Mass low in costovertebral angle or obscured by overlying bone.

Heart

- Examinations of intracardiac anatomy are not indicated at this time. Future advances in CT equipment may allow more clinically useful demonstration of cardiac anatomy and physiology.
- Distinction of cardiac (e.g., ventricular aneurysm) from pericardiac (e.g., mediastinal or pulmonary lesion) mass.
- Detection of aortacoronary vein graft occlusion is possible with intravenous contrast medium bolus with third- and fourth-generation scanners.

Major Blood Vessels

- Evaluation and detection of thoracic aortic aneurysms.
- Screening and measurement of abdominal aortic aneurysms when ultrasound fails or is unavailable.
- Detection of intraluminal clots, chronic leakage, and rupture of thoracic and abdominal aneurysms.
- Evaluation of aortoprosthetic disruption.
- Evaluation of suspected infection of synthetic grafts of the major vessels.
- Delineation of relation of major vessels to retroperitoneal tumors, infections, or other abnormalities.
- Demonstration of invasion of vena cava by tumor.

Spine

- Type I examination: No contrast medium. Type II examination: Dilute metrizamide. Type III examination: Concentrated metrizamide instilled originally for conventional myelography with subsequent CT, performed within 4 hours after metrizamide instillation.
- Evaluation (type I) of spinal stenosis to determine extent and specific causes of bony and soft-tissue encroachment.
  - Diffuse spinal stenosis, congenital or acquired.
  - Localized spinal stenosis, associated with degenerative disease or malalignment.
  - Posttraumatic stenosis: detection of fracture fragments or hematoma.
  - Postspinal fusion stenosis: fusion bone overgrowth.
  - Detection of midline or foramenal spurs not seen on plain films.
  - Combined causes including degenerative, iatrogenic, traumatic, infection/tumor, as well as herniations of the nucleus pulposus.
- Evaluation (types I and II) of congenital dysraphic abnormalities (spina bifida, meningomyelocele, meningocele, diastematomyelia).
- Evaluation (type I or II) of spinal cord and/or nerve root masses, usually as secondary procedure to further determine nature and extent of lesion.
- Localization procedure (type I) for CT-guided biopsy or aspiration.
- Evaluation (type I) of nature and extent of boney or paraspinal tumors and inflammatory masses.

---

*Used by permission of the American Journal of Roentgenology.

- Following nondiagnostic conventional myelography (type I or II procedure) using myelogram and/or clinical findings to specify CT level(s).
- Alternative procedure (type I) in situations precluding standard myelography as primary examination (allergic history, mechanical difficulties, emotional factors).

Retroperitoneum

- Detection of primary malignancies such as those of mesenchymal, neural, lymphatic, and embryonic rest origin, melanomas, and benign conditions, such as cysts that may mimic malignancies.
- Staging of nodal and extranodal extension of lymphomas and other types of retroperitoneal metastases from various primary sites (e.g., initial staging or detection of recurrent metastatic testicular tumor).
- Detection of retroperitoneal abscess or hemorrhage (hematoma); localization for needle aspiration.
- Further evaluation when other radiologic studies unexpectedly suggest abnormality, such as deviated ureter by normal retroperitoneal fat.
- Guidance for retroperitoneal biopsy.

Peritoneum

- Detection and differential diagnosis of free or loculated intraperitoneal fluid collections and inflammatory processes.
- Detection of primary or secondary peritoneal masses (neoplasms and abscesses, etc.)
- Guidance for the aspiration of intraperitoneal fluid collections and peritoneal masses.

Liver

- Evaluation of space-occupying lesions.
  - —— Primary and secondary malignant neoplasms and clinically significant benign lesions, such as adenomas, cavernous hemangiomas, and abscesses.
    - — Initial detection; whether liver is primary organ of interest or examined as part of CT evaluation of other suspected abdominal disease, such as pancreatic carcinoma, in which knowledge of associated hepatic lesions is of clinical importance.
    - — Confirmation of the presence or clarification of the nature of hepatic lesion(s) suspected or found on other imaging procedure, such as an inconclusive or nonspecific radionuclide scan.
    - — Differentiation of solid, cystic, inflammatory, and vascular lesions.
    - — Assessment of location, extent, and number of lesions, when such information is of clinical importance.
    - — Guidance for hepatic biopsy and aspiration.
    - — Assessment of response to nonoperative therapy.
- Evaluation of trauma.
  - —— Detection of hepatic laceration and intrahepatic and subcapsular hematoma, and determination of extent of injury in cases of blunt or penetrating trauma.
- Evaluation of diffuse liver disease.
  - —— CT currently of limited value, but may be useful in specific circumstances, such as detection of fatty infiltration of the liver and conditions of excessive iron deposition (hemochromatosis) and glycogen storage disease in children.

Spleen

- Detection and estimation of age of subcapsular hematoma.
- Detection of intrasplenic mass and differentiation of solid, cystic, and inflammatory lesions.

Pancreas

- Evaluation for possible mass lesion.
  - —— Detection of primary tumor and its extent.
  - —— Search for primary lesion in patient with distant metastases.
  - —— Evaluation of jaundiced patient.
  - —— Evaluation of suspected pancreatitis.
  - —— Evaluation of patient with possible upper abdominal masses.
  - —— Serial assessment of regression or persistence of tumor during and after therapy.
- Differentiation of pancreatic from parapancreatic mass.
  - —— Distinction among solid, cystic, vascular, inflammatory, calcified, and fatty lesions.
- Detection of complications of acute or subacute pancreatitis.
  - —— Detection of pseudocysts, their number, size, and extent.
  - —— Serial assessment of pseudocyst following medical or surgical management.
  - —— Detection of abscess: determination of size and extent.
- Guidance of percutaneous pancreatic biopsy and aspiration procedures.

Kidneys

- Evaluation of kidneys when excretory urography or angiography is contraindicated by risk of serious reaction to contrast medium.
- Evaluation of renal mass or suspected mass detected on another imaging procedure.
  - —— Differentiation of an anatomic variant from a pathologic process.
  - —— Differentiation of a benign fluid-filled cyst from a cyst and/or solid renal mass.
  - —— Determination of the extent of renal neoplasm before and after treatment.
- Evaluation of selected patients, suspected clinically of renal neoplasm, when excretory urogram is negative.
- Evaluation of juxtarenal (para- or perirenal) lesions seen or suspected on excretory urography.
  - —— Differentiation of anatomic variant from pathologic process.
  - —— Determination of the cause, location, and extent of a lesion.
- Evaluation of urographic nonfunctioning kidney(s).
  - —— Assessment of size, outline, and parenchymal thickness.
  - —— Detection of obstruction, determination of site, cause, and extent of disease process.
  - —— Documentation of congenital absence.
  - —— Detection of minimally calcified renal calculi not demonstrated by conventional techniques.
- Determination of cause of renal and perirenal calcification.
- Assessment of extent of renal trauma.
- Guidance for antegrade nephrostomy, renal biopsy, or mass aspiration.

Gallbladder

- CT is not indicated at this time unless oral and intravenous cholecystography and ultrasonography are indeterminate or unobtainable.

Biliary Tree

- Differentiation of obstructive from nonobstructive jaundice.
- Determination of site and etiology of obstruction.
- Determination of etiology of obstruction.

Gastrointestinal Tract

- CT is useful in the assessment of extent or recurrence of tumor or tumorlike condition into the mesentery or adjacent organs. CT is not currently indicated for the detection of mucosal lesions.

Adrenal Gland

- Evaluation of patients with biochemical evidence of adrenal hyperfunction.
- Evaluation of patients with suspicion of adrenal mass found on conventional radiographic examination.
- Guidance for adrenal biopsy.

Uterus and Ovaries

- Evaluation of mass detected by clinical examination, after positive biopsy, after failure of ultrasound examination, or when strong clinical suspicion exists for a mass lesion.
- Evaluation of primary tumor and its extent of spread; and evaluation of secondary tumor.
- Differentiation of solid, cystic, inflammatory, vascular, or fatty masses.
- Guidance for uterine and ovarian biopsy.

Bladder, Ureters, Prostate, and Seminal Vesicles

- Evaluation of primary and secondary tumor, including extent of tumor.

- Differentiation of solid, cystic, inflammatory, vascular, or fatty tumors.
- Detection of obstructing, minimally calcified ureteral calculi not detected by conventional studies.
- Guidance for biopsy.

Pelvic Bones

- Evaluation of bone lesions and accompanying soft tissue extent.
- Guidance for biopsy.

Musculoskeletal System

- Evaluation of selected patients with known or suspected primary bone tumors.
- Evaluation of patients with suspected recurrence of bone tumors.
- Evaluation of patients with suspected but indefinite signs of skeletal metastases when conventional studies fail to clarify.
- Evaluation of joint abnormalities difficult to detect by conventional methods.
- Evaluation of patients with soft tissue tumors, either known or suspected to confirm presence and determine extent.
- Guidance for biopsy.

Therapy Planning and Followup

- Definition of cross-sectional anatomy and attenuation coefficients of bone and soft tissue in tumor-bearing areas for the purpose of planning radiation therapy.
- Provision of baseline prior to radiation therapy and chemotherapy from which effectiveness of these treatment modalities can be judged.
- Conformance as part of an established and acceptable follow-up protocol.
- Evaluation of signs and symptoms suggesting progression, recurrence, or failure of therapy.

Foreign Body Localization

- In chest and abdomen when other traditional imaging techniques provide insufficient information.

CT INDEX

Numbers in *italics* indicate illustrations.
Numbers followed by t indicate tables.